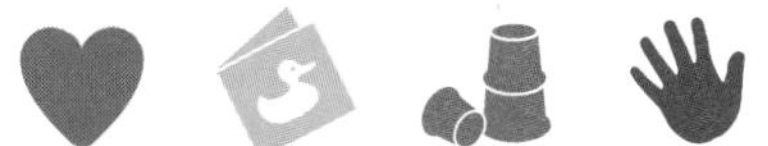

California Infant/Toddler Learning & Development Foundations

California Department of Education
and
WestEd Center for Child and Family Studies

Sacramento, 2009

Publishing Information

The *California Infant/Toddler Learning and Development Foundations* was developed by the Child Development Division, California Department of Education, and WestEd Center for Child and Family Studies. It was edited by Faye Ong, working in cooperation with Tom Cole, Consultant, Quality Improvement Office. It was prepared for printing by the staff of CDE Press: the cover and interior design were created and prepared by Juan D. Sanchez; typesetting was done by Jeannette Reyes. It was published by the Department, 1430 N Street, Sacramento, CA 95814-5901. It was distributed under the provisions of the Library Distribution Act and *Government Code* Section 11096.

ISBN 978-0-8011-1693-3

Notice

The guidance in the *California Infant/Toddler Learning and Development Foundations* is not binding on local educational agencies or other entities. Except for the statutes, regulations, and court decisions that are referenced herein, the document is exemplary, and compliance with it is not mandatory. (See *Education Code* Section 33308.5.)

Contents

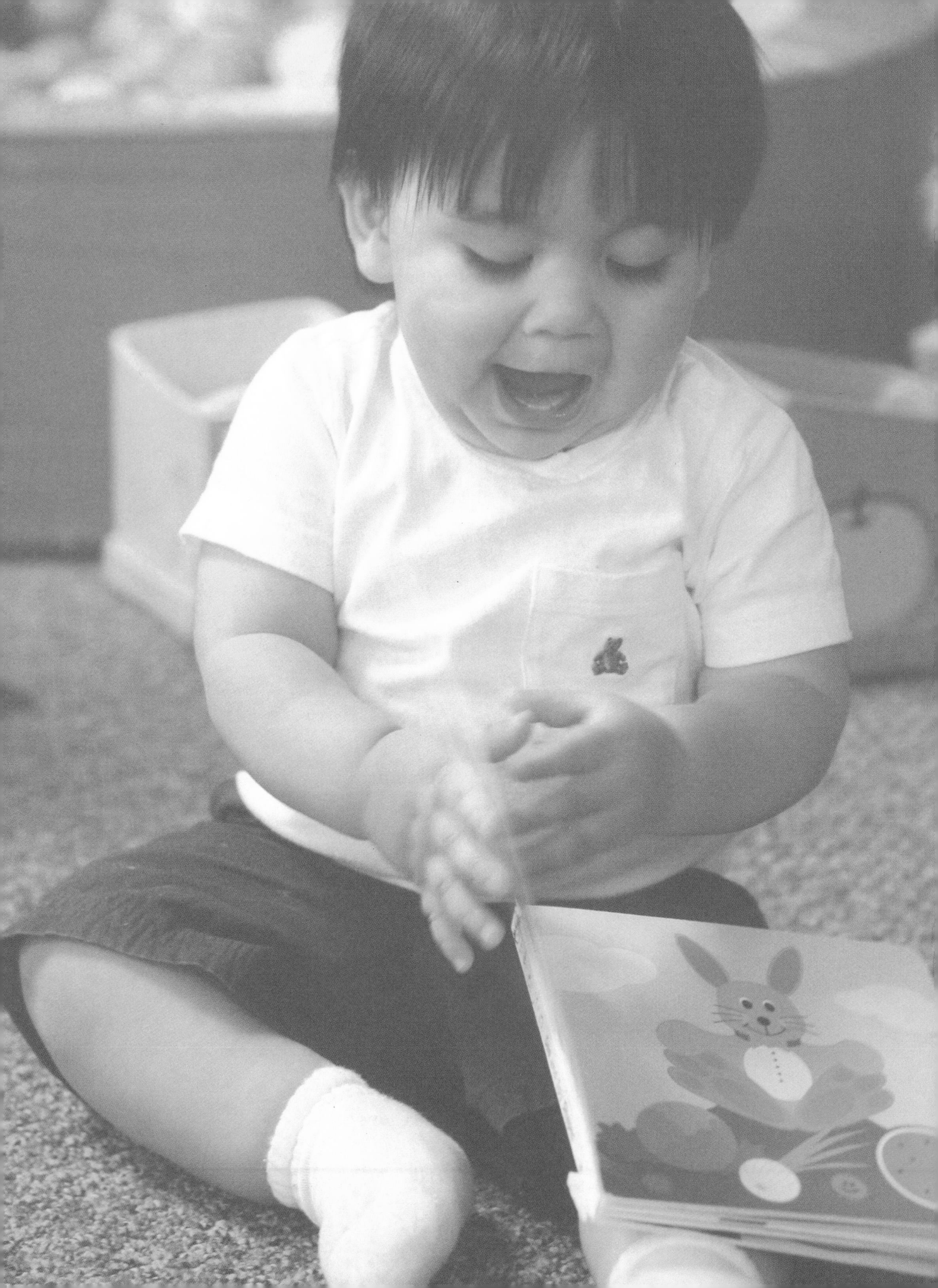

A Message from the State Superintendent of Public Instruction

I am delighted to present the *California Infant/Toddler Learning and Development Foundations*, a publication I believe will contribute to providing high-quality care and education for our youngest children.

The first three years are a crucial time of development. Research on brain development indicates that the brains of infants and toddlers are twice as active as those of adults. By the time children reach the age of three, they have become competent in at least one language, formed a sense of self, learned about basic concepts such as cause-and-effect and quantity, and developed numerous large- and small-muscle skills.

More than half of California's infants and toddlers are cared for in child care centers, in family child care homes, and by relatives or neighbors outside the home. Research shows that good care and education contribute to children's social-emotional, language, cognitive, and perceptual and motor development. High-quality infant/toddler programs provide children with caring relationships, environments, and materials that enrich learning and development. Those programs also develop partnerships with families to connect children's home experiences with experiences in the infant/toddler setting. Partnerships with families are the cornerstone of culturally sensitive care, which is critically important for children's social-emotional well-being and overall learning. With a goal of ensuring that all infant/toddler programs in California offer high-quality care, the California Department of Education collaborated with leading early childhood educators and researchers to develop these learning and development foundations.

The foundations focus on four domains: social-emotional development, language development, cognitive development, and perceptual and motor development. The foundations provide a comprehensive understanding of young children's learning and development during the first three years of life.

It is my hope that these foundations will help all California infant/toddler programs to offer developmentally appropriate and supportive care for our youngest children. By fostering the learning and development described in this publication, infant/toddler care professionals will contribute to children's well-being and lay the foundation for children's future success.

Jack O'Connell

JACK O'CONNELL
State Superintendent of Public Instruction

Acknowledgments

The following people contributed to this publication or helped to develop the ideas:

Panel of Experts

Marc Bornstein, National Institute of Child Health and Human Development
Linda Brault, Sonoma State University
Deborrah Bremond, Alameda County Children and Families Commission
Vera Guttierez-Clellan, San Diego State University
Christopher Lonigan, Florida State University
Tammy Mann, Zero to Three
Lucia Palacios, Los Angeles Universal Preschool
Jeree Pawl, Clinical Psychologist
Todd Risley, University of Alaska
Ross Thompson, University of California, Davis
Marlene Zepeda, California State University, Los Angeles

WestEd, Center for Child and Family Studies

Content development:
Ron Lally, Program Codirector
Peter Mangione, Program Codirector
Charlotte Tilson, Senior Program Associate
Cathy Tsao, Senior Program Associate
Sara Webb-Schmitz, Program Associate
Osnat Zur, Senior Program Associate

Research assistance:
Amy Schustz-Alvarez, Program Assistant
Katie Monahan, Program Assistant
Teresa Ragsdale, Program Assistant

University of California, Berkeley Berkeley Evaluation and Assessment Research Center

Stephen Moore, Center Associate Director
Mark Wilson, Center Director; Professor, UC Berkeley

California Department of Education

Meredith Cathcart, Consultant, Special Education Division
Tom Cole, Consultant, Child Development Division
Cecelia Fisher-Dahms, Administrator, Quality Improvement Office
Michael Jett, Former Director, Child Development Division
Camille Maben, Director, Child Development Division
Anthony Monreal, Deputy Superintendent, Curriculum and Instruction Branch
Mary Smithberger, Consultant, Child Development Division
Gwen Stephens, Former Assistant Director, Child Development Division
Maria Trejo, Administrator, Child Development Division

Note: The names and affiliations of individuals were current at the time of the development of this publication.

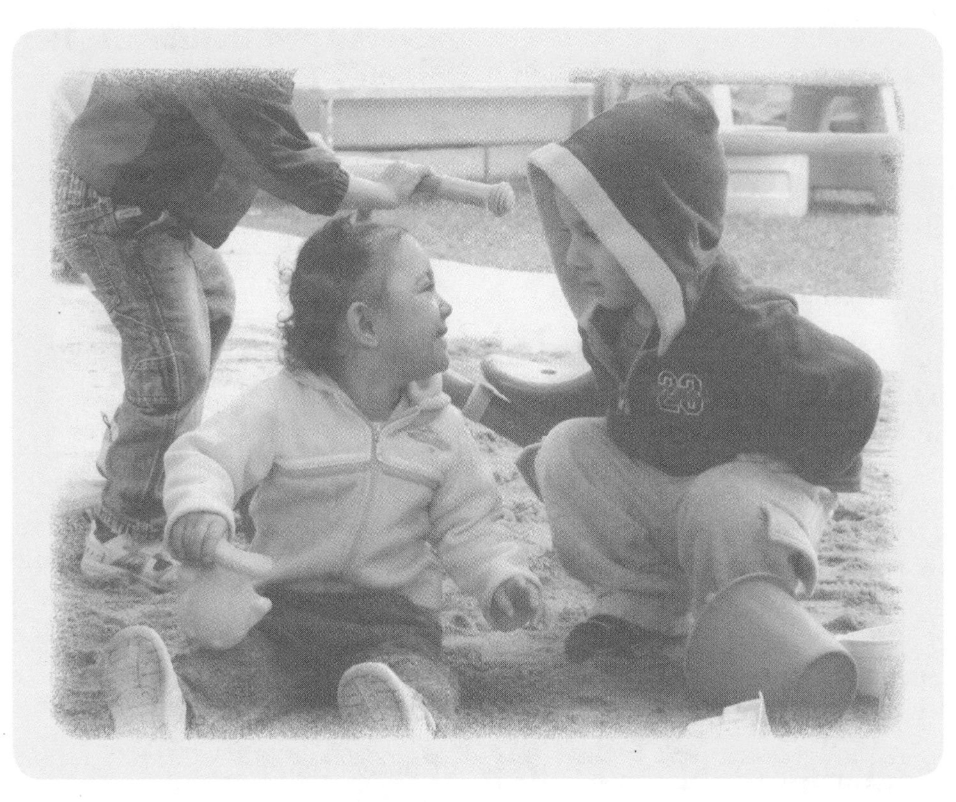

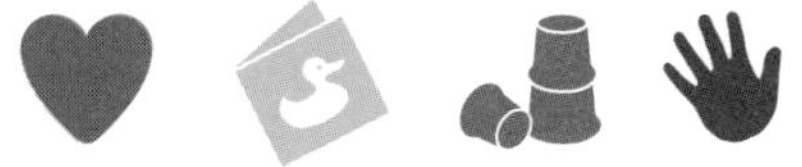

Introduction

The *California Infant/Toddler Learning and Development Foundations* represents part of the California Department of Education's (CDE's) comprehensive effort to strengthen young children's learning and development through high-quality early care and education. The foundations describe competencies infants and toddlers typically attain during the birth-to-three-year period. In order to make developmental progress, young children need appropriate nurturing. Both supportive home environments and high-quality early care and education programs can facilitate children's attainment of the competencies specified in the foundations by providing safe environments and an emotionally secure base for active, playful exploration and experimentation.

During the infant/toddler years, all children depend on responsive, secure relationships to develop and learn. As stated in the CDE's *Infant/Toddler Learning and Development Program Guidelines* (2007), high-quality programs offer infants and toddlers primary relationships in small groups. Such programs provide personalized care that reflects consideration for individual differences among children. Programs also develop partnerships with children's families to connect children's experiences at home with their experiences in the infant/toddler program. These partnerships with families are the cornerstone of culturally sensitive care. Connections with children's early cultural and linguistic experiences are critically important for their social-emotional well-being, the development of their identity, and learning. In addition, children may have a special need that requires particular accommodations and adaptations. To serve all children, infant/toddler programs must work to provide appropriate conditions for each child and individually assist each child's movement along a pathway of healthy learning and development.

Over 20 states have either developed infant/toddler standards documents or are in the process of doing so. Many of them have sought to align infant/toddler standards with preschool learning standards. Because both infant/toddler and preschool foundations in California cover a broad range of learning and development domains, the term *foundations* is used rather than *standards*. This term was selected to convey that learning across all developmental domains builds young children's readiness for school. In essence, the foundations pertain to young children's current and long-term developmental progress. This focus is consonant with the position of the National Association for the Education of Young Children (NAEYC) and the National Association of Early Childhood Specialists in State Departments of Education (NAECS/SDE) on early learning standards. As the position statement sets forth, "Early childhood is a distinct period of life that has value in itself as well as creating the foundations for later years" (NAEYC and NAECS/SDE position statement 2002, 3).

In California, priority has been placed on aligning the infant/toddler learning and development foundations with the preschool learning foundations in four major domains:

- Social-emotional development
- Language development
- Cognitive development
- Perceptual and motor development

The domains represent crucial areas of early learning and development that contribute to young children's readiness for school (National Research Council and Institute of Medicine 2000; NAEYC and NAESC/SDE 2002). The foundations present key concepts in each domain and provide an overview of development in that domain. Young children can be considered from the perspective of one domain, such as social-emotional development or language development. Yet, when taking an in-depth look at a single domain, one needs to keep in mind that learning, for young children, is usually an integrated experience. For example, an infant may make a cognitive discovery about cause-and-effect while making the connection that a cry leads to a comforting response from an adult.

The foundations developed for each of these domains are based on research and evidence from practice. Suggestions of expert practitioners and examples illustrate the foundations. The purpose is to promote understanding of early learning and development and guide efforts to support the development and well-being of infants and toddlers.

Overview of the Foundations

The foundations for each of the four domains are listed in this section.

Social-Emotional Development Domain. The social-emotional development domain covers the following foundations:

- *Interactions with Adults:* The child's developing ability to respond to social cues from adults and engage in back-and-forth social exchanges with adults
- *Relationships with Adults:* The child's development of close relationships with adults who provide consistent nurturance
- *Interactions with Peers:* The child's developing ability to respond to social overtures from peers, engage in back-and-forth interaction with other children, and, ultimately, to engage in cooperative play with other children.
- *Relationships with Peers:* The child's development of relationships with certain peers through interactions over time
- *Identity of Self in Relation to Others:* The child's developing concept of self as an individual who

operates within social relationships

- *Recognition of Ability:* The child's developing understanding of the ability to take action to influence the immediate social and physical environments
- *Expression of Emotion:* The child's developing ability to communicate various emotions through facial expressions, movements, gestures, sounds, or words
- *Empathy:* The child's developing ability to share in the emotional experiences of others
- *Emotion Regulation:* The child's developing ability to manage or regulate emotional responses with and without assistance from adults
- *Impulse Control:* The child's developing capacity to wait for needs to be met, to inhibit behavior, and to act according to social expectations, including safety rules
- *Social Understanding:* The child's developing understanding of the responses, communication, emotional expressions, and actions of other people

The many competencies covered by the social-emotional development foundations underscore the prominence of this domain during the first three years of life. The emotional security that infants seek to develop with others and their ability to interact effectively with both adults and other children support their learning and development in all domains.

Language Development Domain. The language development foundations cover the following competencies:

- *Receptive Language:* The child's developing ability to understand words and increasingly complex utterances
- *Expressive Language:* The child's developing ability to produce the sounds of language, and speak with an increasingly expansive vocabulary and use increasingly complex utterances
- *Communication Skills and Knowledge:* The child's developing ability to communicate nonverbally and verbally
- *Interest in Print:* The child's developing interest in engaging with print in books and in the environment

Many early childhood experts consider language development to be one of the greatest accomplishments in the first three years of life. There are many specific milestones and dimensions of language development, such as phonology and syntax. As to practice, the four foundations provide a level of detail that is accessible to families and infant care teachers seeking to enhance children's early language development and communication.

Cognitive Development Domain. The following foundations make up the cognitive development domain:

- *Cause-and-Effect:* The child's developing understanding that one event or action brings about another
- *Spatial Relationships:* The child's developing understanding of how things move and fit in space

- *Problem Solving:* The child's developing ability to engage in a purposeful effort to reach a goal or to determine how something works
- *Imitation:* The child's developing capacity to mirror, repeat, and practice the actions of others, either immediately or at a later time
- *Memory:* The child's developing ability to store and later retrieve information.
- *Number Sense:* The child's developing understanding of number or quantity
- *Classification:* The child's developing ability to group, sort, categorize, and form expectations based on the attributes of objects and people
- *Symbolic Play:* The child's developing ability to use actions, objects, or ideas to represent other actions, objects, or ideas
- *Attention Maintenance:* The child's developing ability to attend to people and things while interacting with others or exploring the environment and play materials
- *Understanding of Personal Care Routines:* The child's developing ability to understand personal care routines and participate in them

As the above list suggests, the foundations for the cognitive development domain cover a broad range of knowledge and skills. For infants and toddlers, these various competencies are interwoven and develop together. As children move out of the birth-to-three period, some of the cognitive competencies become differentiated and can be aligned with traditional preschool content domains such as mathematics and science. In effect, infants' and toddlers' playful exploration and experimentation in the cognitive domain represent an early manifestation of mathematical and scientific reasoning and problem solving.

Perceptual and Motor Development Domain. Infants' and toddlers' perceptual and motor competencies are receiving increasing attention in research and practice. The perceptual and motor development foundations are defined as follows:

- *Perceptual Development:* The child's developing ability to become aware of the immediate social and physical environments through the senses
- *Gross Motor:* The child's developing ability to move and coordinate large muscles
- *Fine Motor:* The child's developing ability to move and coordinate small muscles

Infant/toddler programs can foster children's perceptual and motor learning and development through environments that offer safe and appropriate physical challenges.

Organization of the Foundations

The publication begins with a chapter that focuses on the first four months of life. Separate foundations in each domain were not written for the first four months because every aspect of early development relates to all domains simultaneously. Although development during the first four months is undifferentiated, it has a profound influence on subsequent development in every domain. The chapter on the early months highlights the inborn behaviors that enable children to orient toward adults and begin to communicate needs. At the same time, the chapter describes how, right from the beginning of life, children are "active participants in their own development, reflecting the intrinsic human drive to explore and master one's environment" (National Research Council and Institute of Medicine 2000, 1).

For each of the 28 foundations, a description is specified at three points of development: at around eight months of age, at around 18 months of age, and at around 36 months of age. In addition, behaviors are listed that lead to the level of competency described for each of those three age levels. The behaviors leading up to an age level reflect the ongoing change that occurs during each age period. At around eight months of age, 18 months of age, and 36 months of age, children move to a different way of functioning and have different developmental needs. For most foundations, the change from one age level (from eight months to 18 months or from 18 months old to 36 months) is quite pronounced. The foundations are designed to give a general sense of development at these three points along the developmental continuum. The subtleties of individual children's developmental progress at any given time are presented in the CDE's Desired Results Developmental Profile (DRDP) (2005). This teacher observation tool for infants and toddlers shows five or six developmental levels spanning the birth-to-three age range for outcomes that will be aligned to the foundations. When alignment of the DRDP to the infant/toddler foundations is complete, the DRDP will provide additional detail about the developmental progression of a foundation.

For each foundation at each of the three age levels, broad information on infant development summarizes children's competencies. Together, the three descriptions define the developmental progression of a foundation. Underneath each description are examples of possible ways that children may demonstrate a foundation in a particular age range. The diversity of examples gives a sense of the variation among infants and toddlers. A foundation for a particular child should be considered on the basis of how the child functions in different contexts—at home, in child care, and in the community. An individual child may not function like any of the examples listed under a foundation, yet she may already be able to demonstrate the level of competency described by that foundation. The examples suggest the varieties of contexts in which children may show competencies reflected in the foundations. Infant care teachers often think of alternative examples when they reflect on how a particular foundation applies to the young children in their care.

Guiding Principles

Several guiding principles influenced the creation of the infant/toddler learning and development foundations. These principles stem from both developmental theory and research and from best practice in the infant/toddler care field.

1. The family and its culture and language play a central role in early learning and development.

2. Infancy is a unique stage of life that is important in its own right. Development in infancy can be described by three age periods—birth to eight months, eight months to 18 months, and 18 months to 36 months. Each age period is distinct, although there is often overlap from one to the next.
3. Infants and toddlers are competent yet vulnerable at every stage of development. Nurturing relationships provide the foundation for emotional security and optimal learning and development.
4. Emotions drive early learning. Infants and toddlers are active, curious learners who are internally driven to interact with social and physical environments. Infants and toddlers learn in a holistic way rather than one domain at a time.
5. Early development includes both quantitative and qualitative change. With quantitative shifts, the infant extends or adds competencies to similar existing competencies. With qualitative shifts, the infant combines new knowledge and abilities with existing knowledge and abilities to function in a different and more complex way.
6. Early development reflects an interplay of differentiation and integration. For example, young infants typically use their mouths to explore all objects to learn about them (less differentiated behavior), whereas older children mainly use their mouth to taste or explore different kinds of food (more differentiated behavior). An example of integration is that older children may be able to engage in several behaviors such as talking, walking, and carrying an object simultaneously (more integrated behavior), whereas younger children may need to focus all of their energies on doing one behavior at a time (less integrated behavior).

Those principles apply to the foundations, curriculum planning, and assessment practices aligned to the foundations.

Universal Design for Learning

These foundations support infant/toddler programs in the effort to foster the learning and development of all young children in California, including children with disabilities or other special needs. In some cases, infants and toddlers with disabilities or other special needs will reveal their developmental progress in alternative ways. It is important to provide opportunities for children to follow different pathways to learning. Therefore, the infant/toddler learning and development foundations incorporate a concept known as universal design for learning.

Developed by the Center for Applied Special Technology (CAST), universal design for learning is based on the realization that children learn in different ways. In today's diverse infant/toddler programs, making the environment, play materials, activities, and experiences accessible to all children is critical to successful learning. Universal design is not a single approach that will accommodate everyone; rather, it refers to providing multiple approaches to learning in order to meet the needs of diverse learners. Universal design provides for multiple means of representation, multiple means of engagement, and multiple means of expression (CAST 2007). "Multiple means of representation" refers to providing information in a variety of ways so the learning needs of all children are met. "Multiple means of expression" refers to allowing children to use alternative ways to communicate or demonstrate what they know or what they are feeling. "Multiple means of engagement" refers to providing choices within the setting or program that facilitate learning by building on children's interests.

The examples in the infant/toddler learning and development foundations have been worded to portray multiple means of representation, expression, and engagement. A variety of examples are provided for each foundation, and inclusive words are used to describe children's behavior. For example, rather than stating "The child looks at an object" or "The child listens to a person," the more inclusive wording of "A child attends to an object" or "The child attends to a person" is used.

When reading each foundation, an infant care teacher needs to consider the means by which a child with a disability or other special need might best acquire information and act competently. To best meet a child's needs, a parent and an early intervention specialist or related service provider are vitally important resources.

The Foundations and Infant/Toddler Care and Education in California

The CDE's learning and development foundations are at the center of California's infant/toddler learning and development system. The foundations describe how children develop and what they learn and are designed to illuminate the competencies that infants and toddlers need for later success. Together the components of the infant/toddler learning and development system provide information and resources to help early childhood professionals support infants, toddlers, and their families.

- In the *Infant/Toddler Learning and Development Program Guidelines* there are recommendations for setting up environments, providing infants a secure base for learning and exploration, selecting appropriate materials, and planning and implementing learning opportunities.
- The Infant/Toddler Desired Results Developmental Profile (described earlier in this chapter) is an observational assessment instrument that allows teachers to document individual children's developmental progress.
- The infant/toddler curriculum framework will provide general guidance on the kinds of environments and interactions that support learning and development.
- The Program for Infant/Toddler Care is a comprehensive approach to professional development that provides infant/toddler professionals with opportunities to become informed about the infant/toddler learning and development foundations and other components of California's infant/toddler system.

As a unifying element of California's infant/toddler learning and development system, the foundations offer a common language for infant/toddler program directors, teachers, and families to reflect on children's developmental progress and plan experiences that support children's learning and development during the first three years of life.

Professional development is another key component in fostering infant/toddler learning and development. Professionals now have opportunities to become informed: through the infant/toddler learning and development foundations, the CDE's *Infant/Toddler Learning and Development Program Guidelines*, the CDE's Desired Results Developmental Profile (DRDP), and the Program for Infant/Toddler Care (the comprehensive approach to training collaboratively developed by the CDE and WestEd). The foundations can become a unifying element for both preservice and in-service professional development efforts. For infant/toddler programs, directors and teachers can use the foundations as a basis to reflect on children's developmental progress and to plan experiences that support children's learning and development from birth to three years. The foundations are designed to provide infant care teachers with knowledge of the competencies necessary during the first three years of a child's life and later on in preschool and school.

References

California Department of Education (CDE). 2007. *Infant/Toddler Learning and Development Program Guidelines.* Sacramento: CDE Press.

Center for Applied Special Technology (CAST). 2007. *Universal Design for Learning.* http://www.cast.org/udl/ (accessed June 8, 2007).

National Association for the Education of Young Children (NAEYC) and Association of Early Childhood Specialists in State Departments of Education (NAECS/SDE). 2002. *Early Learning Standards: Creating the Conditions for Success.* Washington, DC: National Association for the Education of Young Children.

National Research Council and Institute of Medicine. 2000. *From Neurons to Neighborhoods: The Science of Early Childhood Development.* Committee on Integrating the Science of Early Childhood Development. Edited by J. Shonkoff and D. Phillips. Washington, DC: National Academy Press.

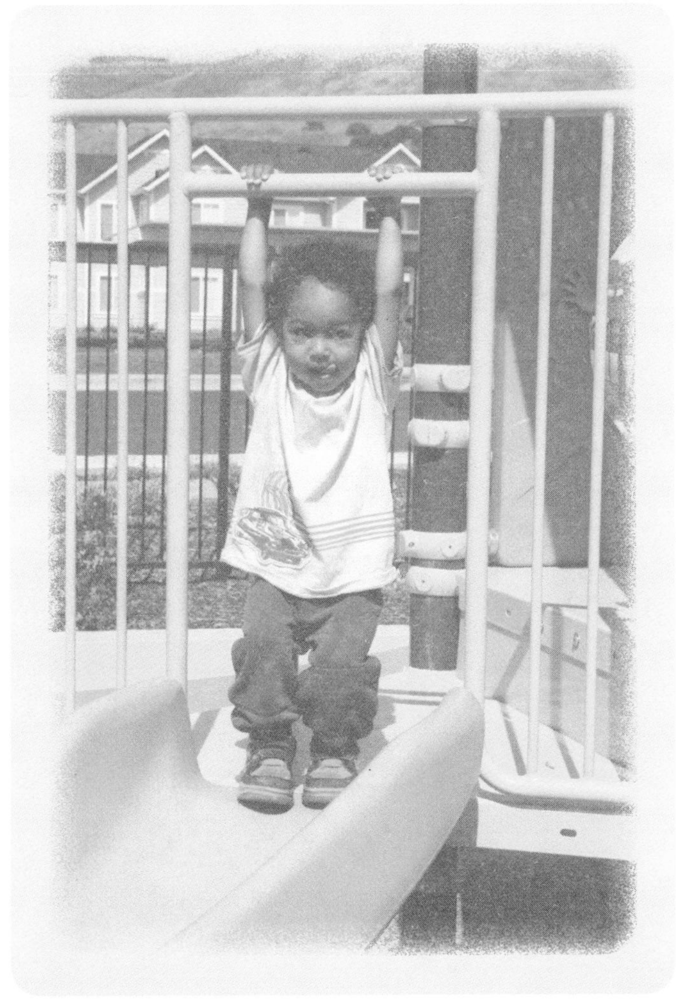

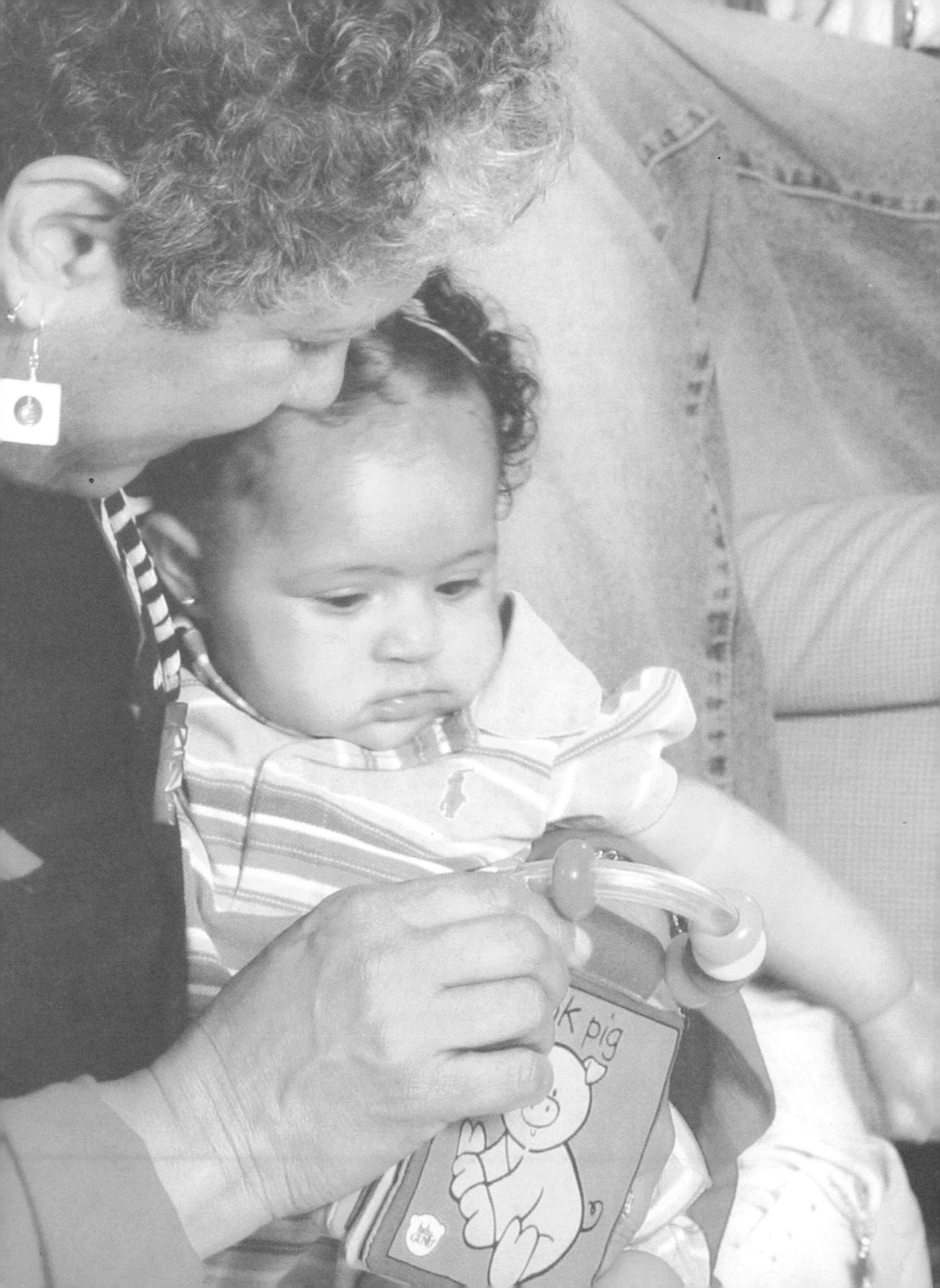

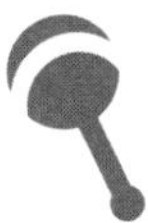

The Early Months

With regard to very young infants, Magda Gerber commented:

> Everything they see, they hear, they feel, they touch is new. . . . They are adapting to all that newness, adapting to their inner physiological needs, which are plenty. . . . A very young baby is busy being a very young baby. (*Respectfully Yours* 1988, 5)

During the first four months of life, babies begin to engage the world and the people in it (*Advances in Applied Developmental Psychology* 1995). Infants' motivation to explore and communicate drives them to move their bodies, focus their attention, and send and receive signals—the basis for development and learning in all domains. These early behaviors mark the start of a child's developmental progress (Emde 1990).

Young babies seek relationships and build knowledge. They actively explore what they can do with their bodies, people close to them, and the environment. They are not empty vessels waiting to be filled with information, but rather "active participants in their own development, reflecting the intrinsic human drive to explore and master one's environment" (National Research Council and Institute of Medicine 2000, 1). Their active engagement with the social and physical world works hand in hand with the care they receive from adults, especially when the adults are responsive to them.

The Newborn

From birth babies learn to connect internal sensory experiences to movements of their bodies. They repeatedly attend to sensory experiences and explore movements they can make. In doing so, they make discoveries about their bodies—how to use their head, eyes, mouth, arms, and legs. Young babies also use their senses to learn about people and things.

Much of the earliest learning of typically developing infants comes through their use of vision. Even very young babies watch their mothers' and other adults' faces intently, and what they see influences their behavior (Schore 1994). Babies also seek eye-to-eye connection with adults. They use their eyes to both send messages and to gain information. In the first months of life, babies are aroused by social engagement and quieted by mutual gazing experiences (Stern 1977). Both the arousal and the calming positively affect the development of the child's brain and stimulate the onset of self-regulation (Emde 1988). Reading and understanding babies' gazes and showing interest and warmth by gazing in return benefit the children greatly.

Babies develop quickly by extending their abilities in all domains and by creating more complex ways of relating to people and things. They send messages to adults in various ways and come to expect responses from adults. For example, when looking into the faces of adults, infants may see enlarged dilated pupils—a common sign of interest and pleasure—and, in response, they smile more (Hess 1975). Spitz and Wolfe (1946) observed that newborns exhibit three distinct reactions to internal and external stimuli:

- Quiescence (a calm state)
- Undifferentiated excitement (a general response to pleasurable stimuli)
- "Unpleasure"

By the end of the first month the "unpleasure" differentiates or branches out into signs of displeasure and signs of distress.[1] One-month-olds show signs of displeasure when they dislike an experience and signs of distress when they experience discomfort or pain. By the second or third month, undifferentiated excitement also differentiates or branches out into two types of distinct responses: (1) clear signs of pleasure and (2) positive social responses to people, including the above-mentioned smiling, increased vocalizations, and bodily activity.

The Three- to Four-Month-Old Infant

By three months of age, pathways of hearing and sight are actively shaping in the brain. The developing brain adapts to the messages it receives from the eyes and the ears by either pruning (weakening) or making robust synaptic connections for future functioning.

Pruning of some synaptic connections and strengthening of others can be seen in early language development. Newborns are responsive to the sounds of all human languages. By the age of three to four months, babies are increasingly sensitive and alert to the sounds of the language(s) spoken by adults who care for them and become less attuned to the sounds of other languages.

As infants approach four months, they become increasingly skilled at using a variety of ways to understand and relate to the world around them. They create basic categories, such as things that move and things that do not (Mandler 2004), and start to treat things differently according to attributes such as "hard," "soft," or "sticky." For example, they may change how they hold and grasp things based on the attributes of the objects held. Young infants also try to prolong interesting experiences; then, after doing the same activity for a while and mastering it, they experiment in search of novelty.

Children in the three- to four-month range also show highly differentiated

---

[1] When a reference is made to a specific age, the following qualifying statements always apply: The reference is to developmental age, rather than chronological age. The phrase "at around" always either explicitly or implicitly precedes the stated age, to recognize variation in individual development.

A behavior stated for an age is not strictly based on maturation, but also stems from experience and practice.

social-emotional behavior. By three months, babies have already learned to alter their responses to adults according to how the adults respond to them. For example, when adults acknowledge babies' vocalizations with a smile, a vocal response, or light touch, children increase their vocalizations. The interest of others stimulates the interest of the baby (Crick 1984).

The power children have in relationships, by four months of age, is clearly evident, as is the power that relationships have over them. They are becoming more skilled at reading others' behavior and adapting their own behavior. They are also gaining skills to make themselves increasingly engaging and effective socially. Four-month-olds will:

- Send clear messages.
- Become quiet in anticipation as someone comes near to care for them.
- Seek adults' attention with smiles and laughter.
- Participate in extended back and forth interaction with others.
- Engage in simple social imitation.

Emotionally, infants grow just as rapidly as they grow socially. Compared with younger babies, babies at around four months send clearer emotional messages through varying cries, movements, and facial expressions. They also show pleasure when mastering simple motor tasks such as when they successfully position their bodies for exploration. Positive emotional experiences motivate infants to keep practicing new skills, exploring new possibilities, and learning.

Interpreting and Responding to Early Development

In the first few months, amazing advances occur in infants' development. Starting with basic responses, newborns reach out to the world. Within weeks they come to expect and depend on appropriate responses from those who care for them.

Noticing and responding to key aspects of growth during this rapid developmental period can be challenging. Early behaviors in one developmental domain are often coupled with behaviors in other domains. In addition, many early behaviors may mean several things at the same time. For example, a young baby's cry may simultaneously represent the beginning of communication (language development), a tool for getting needs met (intellectual development), and a way of relating to others (social-emotional development). Or behaviors that look almost identical may have a different meaning at different times. For example, at one time prolonged focus on a person may be an emerging strategy to deepen emotional connections. At another time, this same behavior may be a way to increase understanding of how people move in space. To be in tune with young babies, adults need to know both when a baby wants a social response and when a baby is making a discovery through individual exploration and observation.

Because major changes that occur during the first few months of life are sometimes difficult to identify, one can easily miss them. Yet the advances of the early months are just as important to a young child's healthy development as are the more obvious advances of the eight-month-old and older infant. When adults understand the sucking, clinging, body position, smiling, crying, and gazes of the young baby, they are better able to respond to the baby's needs.

By recognizing and giving appropriate responses to a baby's early developmental achievements, adults offer an incredible gift. Adults communicate that the path the baby is progressively moving along is understood and supported. This communication lays the foundation for the young baby's emerging emotional security and attachment relationships, which are essential for all learning and development throughout the early years.

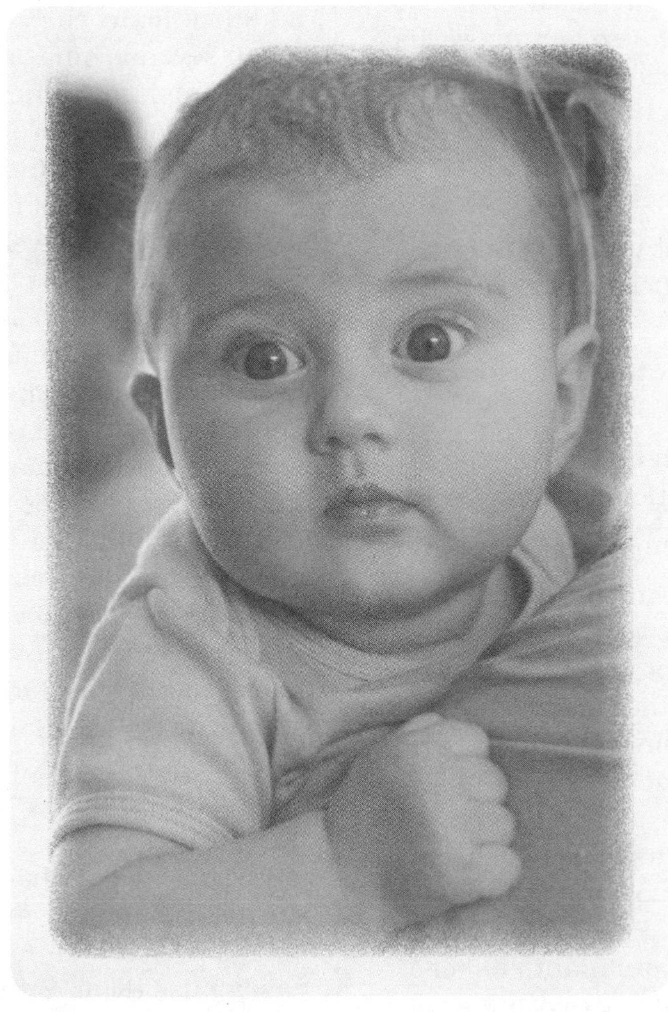

References

Advances in Applied Developmental Psychology: Mastery Motivation: Origins, Conceptualizations, and Applications (Vol. 12). 1995. Edited by R. H. MacTurk and G. A. Morgan. Norwood, NJ: Greenwood Publishing Group.

Crick, F. 1984. "Function of the Thalamic Reticular Complex: The Searchlight Hypothesis," *Proceedings of the National Academy of Sciences of the United States of America,* Vol. 81, 4586–90.

Emde, R. N. 1988. "Development Terminable and Interminable. I. Innate and Motivational Factors from Infancy," *International Journal of Psychoanalysis,* Vol. 69, 23–42.

Hess, E. H. 1975. "The Role of Pupil Size in Communication," *Scientific American,* Vol. 233,110–19.

Mandler, J. M. 2004. *The Foundations of the Mind: Origins of Conceptual Thought.* New York: Oxford University Press.

National Research Council and Institute of Medicine. 2000. *From Neurons to Neighborhoods: The Science of Early Childhood Development.* Committee on Integrating the Science of Early Childhood. Edited by J. Shonkoff and D. Phillips. Washington, DC: National Academies Press.

Respectfully Yours: Magda Gerber's Approach to Professional Infant/Toddler Care (Video magazine). 1988. Sacramento: California Department of Education in collaboration with WestEd Center for Child and Family Studies.

Schore, A. N. 1994. *The Neurobiolgy of Emotional Development.* Hillsdale, NJ: Lawrence Erlbaum Associates.

Spitz, R. A., and K. M. Wolfe. 1946. "The Smiling Response: A Contribution to the Ontogenesis of Social Relation," *Genetic Psychology Monographs,* Vol. 34, 57–125.

Stern, D. N. 1977. *The First Relationship: Infant and Mother.* Cambridge, UK: Harvard University Press.

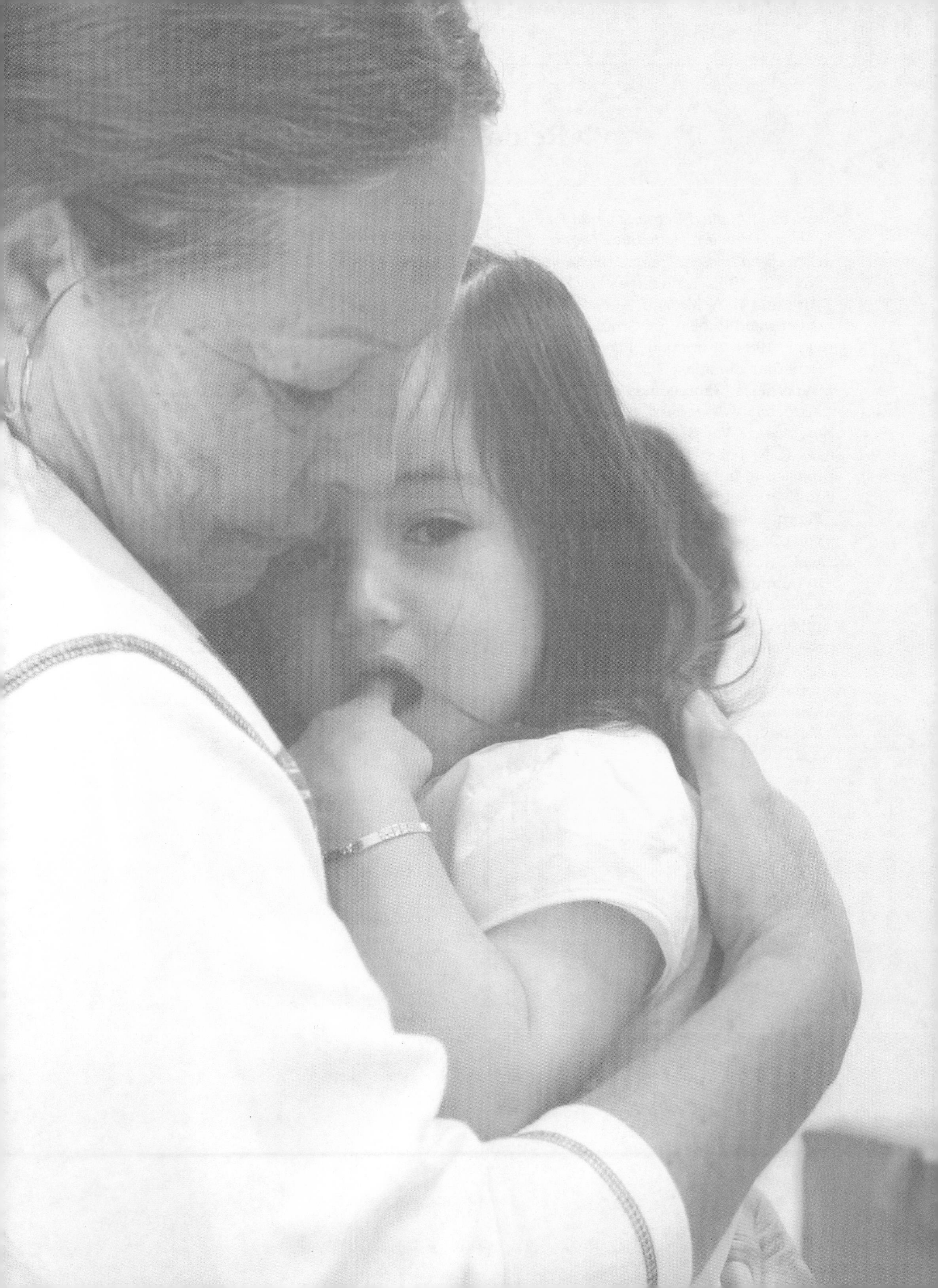

Social-Emotional Development

Social-emotional development includes the child's experience, expression, and management of emotions and the ability to establish positive and rewarding relationships with others (Cohen and others 2005). It encompasses both intra- and interpersonal processes.

> The core features of emotional development include the ability to identify and understand one's own feelings, to accurately read and comprehend emotional states in others, to manage strong emotions and their expression in a constructive manner, to regulate one's own behavior, to develop empathy for others, and to establish and maintain relationships. (National Scientific Council on the Developing Child 2004, 2)

Infants experience, express, and perceive emotions before they fully understand them. In learning to recognize, label, manage, and communicate their emotions and to perceive and attempt to understand the emotions of others, children build skills that connect them with family, peers, teachers, and the community. These growing capacities help young children to become competent in negotiating increasingly complex social interactions, to participate effectively in relationships and group activities, and to reap the benefits of social support crucial to healthy human development and functioning.

Healthy social-emotional development for infants and toddlers unfolds in an interpersonal context, namely that of positive ongoing relationships with familiar, nurturing adults. Young children are particularly attuned to social and emotional stimulation. Even newborns appear to attend more to stimuli that resemble faces (Johnson and others 1991). They also prefer their mothers' voices to the voices of other women (DeCasper and Fifer 1980). Through nurturance, adults support the infants' earliest experiences of emotion regulation (Bronson 2000a; Thompson and Goodvin 2005).

Responsive caregiving supports infants in beginning to regulate their emotions and to develop a sense of predictability, safety, and responsiveness in their social environments. Early relationships are so important to developing infants that research experts have broadly concluded that, in the early years, "nurturing, stable and consistent relationships are the

key to healthy growth, development and learning" (National Research Council and Institute of Medicine 2000, 412). In other words, high-quality relationships increase the likelihood of positive outcomes for young children (Shonkoff 2004). Experiences with family members and teachers provide an opportunity for young children to learn about social relationships and emotions through exploration and predictable interactions. Professionals working in child care settings can support the social-emotional development of infants and toddlers in various ways, including interacting directly with young children, communicating with families, arranging the physical space in the care environment, and planning and implementing curriculum.

Brain research indicates that emotion and cognition are profoundly interrelated processes. Specifically, "recent cognitive neuroscience findings suggest that the neural mechanisms underlying emotion regulation may be the same as those underlying cognitive processes" (Bell and Wolfe 2004, 366). Emotion and cognition work together, jointly informing the child's impressions of situations and influencing behavior. Most learning in the early years occurs in the context of emotional supports (National Research Council and Institute of Medicine 2000). "The rich interpenetrations of emotions and cognitions establish the major psychic scripts for each child's life" (Panksepp 2001). Together, emotion and cognition contribute to attentional processes, decision making, and learning (Cacioppo and Berntson 1999). Furthermore, cognitive processes, such as decision making, are affected by emotion (Barrett and others 2007). Brain structures involved in the neural circuitry of cognition influence emotion and vice versa (Barrett and others 2007). Emotions and social behaviors affect the young child's ability to persist in goal-oriented activity, to seek help when it is needed, and to participate in and benefit from relationships.

Young children who exhibit healthy social, emotional, and behavioral adjustment are more likely to have good academic performance in elementary school (Cohen and others 2005; Zero to Three 2004). The sharp distinction between cognition and emotion that has historically been made may be more of an artifact of scholarship than it is representative of the way these processes occur in the brain (Barrett and others 2007). This recent research strengthens the view that early childhood programs support later positive learning outcomes in all domains by maintaining a focus on the promotion of healthy social emotional development (National Scientific Council on the Developing Child 2004; Raver 2002; Shonkoff 2004).

Interactions with Adults

Interactions with adults are a frequent and regular part of infants' daily lives. Infants as young as three months of age have been shown to be able to discriminate between the faces of unfamiliar adults (Barrera and Maurer 1981). The foundations that describe Interactions with Adults and Relationships with Adults are interrelated. They jointly give a picture of healthy social-emotional development that is based in a supportive social environment established by adults. Children develop the ability to both respond to adults and engage with them first through predictable interactions in close relationships with parents or other caring adults at home and outside the home. Children use and build upon the skills learned through close relationships to interact with less familiar adults in their lives. In interacting with adults, children engage in a wide variety of social exchanges such as establishing contact with a relative or engaging in storytelling with an infant care teacher.

> Quality in early childhood programs is, in large part, a function of the interactions that take place between the adults and children in those programs. These interactions form the basis for the relationships that are established between teachers and children in the classroom or home and are related to children's developmental status. How teachers interact with children is at the very heart of early childhood education (Kontos and Wilcox-Herzog 1997, 11).

Relationships with Adults

Close relationships with adults who provide consistent nurturance strengthen children's capacity to learn and develop. Moreover, relationships with parents, other family members, caregivers, and teachers provide the key context for infants' social-emotional development. These special relationships influence the infant's emerging sense of self and understanding of others. Infants use relationships with adults in many ways: for reassurance that they are safe, for assistance in alleviating distress, for help with emotion regulation, and for social approval or encouragement. Establishing close relationships with adults is related to children's emotional security, sense of self, and evolving understanding of the world around them. Concepts from the literature on attachment may be applied to early childhood settings, in considering the infant care teacher's role in separations and reunions during the day in care, facilitating the child's exploration, providing comfort, meeting physical needs, modeling positive relationships, and providing support during stressful times (Raikes 1996).

Interactions with Peers

In early infancy children interact with each other using simple behaviors such as looking at or touching another child. Infants' social interactions with peers increase in complexity from engaging in repetitive or routine back-and-forth interactions with peers (for example, rolling a ball back and forth) to engaging in cooperative activities such as building a tower of blocks together or acting out different roles during pretend play. Through interactions with peers, infants explore their interest in others and learn about social behavior/social interaction. Interactions with peers provide the context for social learning and problem solving, including the experience of social exchanges, cooperation, turn-taking, and the demonstration of the beginning of empathy. Social interactions with peers also allow older infants to experiment with different roles in small groups and in different situations such as relating to familiar versus unfamiliar children. As noted, the foundations called Interactions with Adults, Relationships with Adults, Interactions with Peers, and Relationships with Peers are interrelated.

Interactions are stepping-stones to relationships. Burk (1996, 285) writes:

> We, as teachers, need to facilitate the development of a psychologically safe environment that promotes positive social interaction. As children interact openly with their peers, they learn more about each other as individuals, and they begin building a history of interactions.

Relationships with Peers

Infants develop close relationships with children they know over a period of time, such as other children in the family child care setting or neighborhood. Relationships with peers provide young children with the opportunity to develop strong social connections. Infants often show a preference for playing and being with friends, as compared with peers with whom they do not have a relationship. Howes' (1983) research suggests that there are distinctive patterns of friendship for the infant, toddler, and preschooler age groups. The three groups vary in the number of friendships, the stability of friendships, and the nature of interaction between friends (for example, the extent to which they involve object exchange or verbal communication).

Identity of Self in Relation to Others

Infants' social-emotional development includes an emerging awareness of self and others. Infants demonstrate this foundation in a number of ways. For example, they can respond to their names, point to their body parts when asked, or name members of their families. Through an emerging understanding of other people in their social environment, children gain an understanding of their roles within their families and communities. They also become aware of their own preferences and characteristics and those of others.

Recognition of Ability

Infants' developing sense of self-efficacy includes an emerging understanding that they can make things happen and that they have particular abilities. Self-efficacy is related to a sense of competency, which has been identified as a basic human need (Connell 1990). The development of children's sense of self-efficacy may be seen in play or exploratory behaviors when they act on an object to produce a result. For example, they pat a musical toy to make sounds come out. Older infants may demonstrate recognition of ability through "I" statements, such as "I did it" or "I'm good at drawing."

Expression of Emotion

Even early in infancy, children express their emotions through facial expressions, vocalizations, and body language. The later ability to use words to express emotions gives young children a valuable tool in gaining the assistance or social support of others (Saarni and others 2006). Temperament may play a role in children's expression of emotion. Tronick (1989, 112) described how expression of emotion is related to emotion regulation and communication between the mother and infant: "the emotional expressions of the infant and the caretaker function to allow them to mutually regulate their interactions . . . the infant and the adult are participants in an affective communication system."

Both the understanding and expression of emotion are influenced by culture. Cultural factors affect children's growing understanding of the meaning of emotions, the developing knowledge of which situations lead to which emotional outcomes, and their learning about which emotions are appropriate to display in which situations (Thompson and Goodvin 2005). Some cultural groups appear to express certain emotions more often than other cultural groups (Tsai, Levenson, and McCoy 2006). In addition, cultural groups vary by which particular emotions or emotional states they value (Tsai, Knutson, and Fung 2006). One study suggests that cultural differences in exposure to particular emotions through storybooks may contribute to young children's preferences for particular emotional states (for example, excited or calm) (Tsai and others 2007).

Young children's expression of positive and negative emotions may play a significant role in their development of social relationships. Positive emotions appeal to social partners and seem to enable relationships to form, while problematic management or expression of negative emotions leads to difficulty in social relationships (Denham and Weissberg 2004). The use of emotion-related words appears to be associated with how likable preschoolers are considered by their peers. Children who use emotion-related words were found to be better-liked by their classmates (Fabes and others 2001). Infants respond more positively to adult vocalizations that have a positive affective tone (Fernald 1993). Social smiling is a developmental process in which neurophysiology and cognitive, social, and emotional factors play a part, seen as a "reflection and constituent of an interactive relationship" (Messinger and Fogel 2007, 329). It appears likely that the experience of positive emotions is a particularly important contributor to emotional well-being and psychological health (Fredrickson 2000, 2003; Panksepp 2001).

Empathy

During the first three years of life, children begin to develop the capacity to experience the emotional or psychological state of another person (Zahn-Waxler and Radke-Yarrow 1990). The following definitions of empathy are found in the research literature: "knowing what another person is feeling," "feeling what another person is feeling," and "responding compassionately to another's distress" (Levenson and Ruef 1992, 234). The concept of empathy reflects the social nature of emotion, as it links the feelings of two or more people (Levenson and Ruef 1992). Since human life is relationship-based, one vitally important function of empathy over the life span is to strengthen social bonds (Anderson and Keltner 2002). Research has shown a correlation between empathy and prosocial behavior (Eisenberg 2000). In particular, prosocial behaviors, such as helping, sharing, and comforting or showing concern for others, illustrate the development of empathy (Zahn-Waxler and others 1992) and how the experience of empathy is thought to be related to the development of moral behavior (Eisenberg 2000). Adults model prosocial/empathic behaviors for infants in various ways. For example, those behaviors are modeled through caring interactions with oth-

ers or through providing nurturance to the infant. Quann and Wien (2006, 28) suggest that one way to support the development of empathy in young children is to create a culture of caring in the early childhood environment: "Helping children understand the feelings of others is an integral aspect of the curriculum of living together. The relationships among teachers, between children and teachers, and among children are fostered with warm and caring interactions."

Emotion Regulation

The developing ability to regulate emotions has received increasing attention in the research literature (Eisenberg, Champion, and Ma 2004). Researchers have generated various definitions of emotion regulation, and debate continues as to the most useful and appropriate way to define this concept (Eisenberg and Spinrad 2004). As a construct, emotion regulation reflects the interrelationship of emotions, cognitions, and behaviors (Bell and Wolfe 2004). Young children's increasing understanding and skill in the use of language is of vital importance in their emotional development, opening new avenues for communicating about and regulating emotions (Campos, Frankel, and Camras 2004) and helping children to negotiate acceptable outcomes to emotionally charged situations in more effective ways. Emotion regulation is influenced by culture and the historical era in which a person lives: cultural variability in regulation processes is significant (Mesquita and Frijda 1992). "Cultures vary in terms of what one is expected to feel, and when, where, and with whom one may express different feelings" (Cheah and Rubin 2003, 3). Adults can provide positive role models of emotion regulation through their behavior and through the verbal and emotional support they offer children in managing their emotions. Responsiveness to infants' signals contributes to the development of emotion regulation. Adults support infants' development of emotion regulation by minimizing exposure to excessive stress, chaotic environments, or over- or understimulation.

Emotion regulation skills are important in part because they play a role in how well children are liked by peers and teachers and how socially competent they are perceived to be (National Scientific Council on the Developing Child 2004). Children's ability to regulate their emotions appropriately can contribute to perceptions of their overall social skills as well as to the extent to which they are liked by peers (Eisenberg and others 1993). Poor emotion regulation can impair children's thinking, thereby compromising their judgment and decision making (National Scientific Council on the Developing Child 2004). At kindergarten entry, children demonstrate broad variability in their ability to self-regulate (National Research Council and Institute of Medicine 2000).

Impulse Control

Children's developing capacity to control impulses helps them adapt to social situations and follow rules. As infants grow, they become increasingly able to exercise voluntary control over behavior such as waiting for needs to be met, inhibiting potentially hurtful behavior, and acting according to social expectations, including safety rules. Group care settings provide many opportunities for children to practice their impulse-control skills. Peer interactions often offer natural opportunities for young children to practice impulse control, as they make progress in learning about cooperative play and sharing. Young children's understanding or lack of understanding of requests made of them may be one factor contributing to their responses (Kaler and Kopp 1990).

Social Understanding

During the infant/toddler years, children begin to develop an understanding of the responses, communication, emotional expression, and actions of other people. This development includes infants' understanding of what to expect from others, how to engage in back-and-forth social interactions, and which social scripts are to be used for which social situations. "At each age, social cognitive understanding contributes to social competence, interpersonal sensitivity, and an awareness of how the self relates to other individuals and groups in a complex social world" (Thompson 2006, 26). Social understanding is particularly important because of the social nature of humans and human life, even in early infancy (Wellman and Lagattuta 2000). Recent research suggests that infants' and toddlers' social understanding is related to how often they experience adult communication about the thoughts and emotions of others (Taumoepeau and Ruffman 2008).

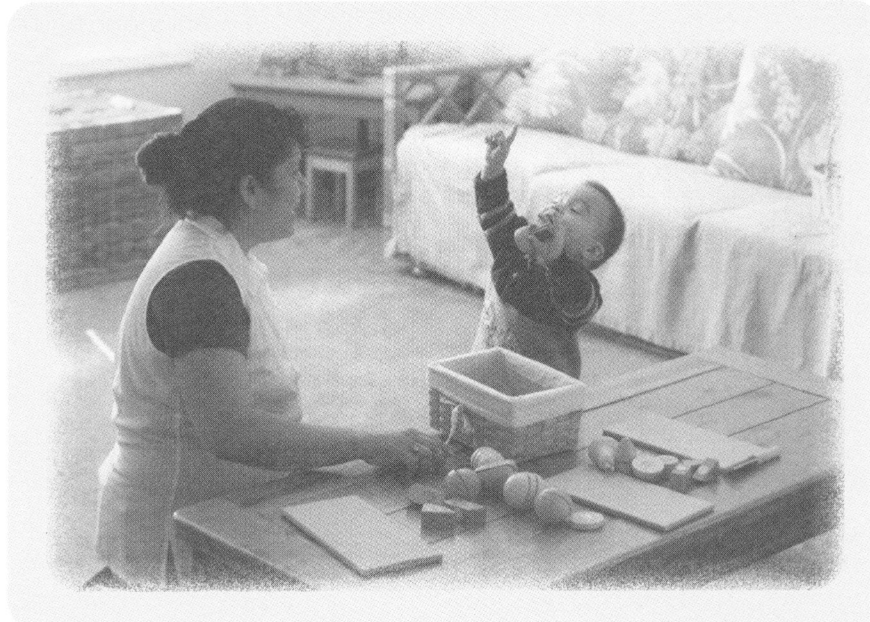

Foundation: Interactions with Adults

The developing ability to respond to and engage with adults

8 months	*18 months*	*36 months*
At around eight months of age, children purposefully engage in reciprocal interactions and try to influence the behavior of others. Children may be both interested in and cautious of unfamiliar adults. (7 mos.; Lamb, Bornstein, and Teti 2002, 340) (8 mos.; Meisels and others 2003, 16)	At around 18 months of age, children may participate in routines and games that involve complex back-and-forth interaction and may follow the gaze of the infant care teacher to an object or person. Children may also check with a familiar infant care teacher when uncertain about something or someone. (18 mos.; Meisels and others 2003, 33)	At around 36 months of age, children interact with adults to solve problems or communicate about experiences or ideas. (California Department of Education 2005, 6; Marvin and Britner 1999, 60).
For example, the child may:	**For example, the child may:**	**For example, the child may:**
• Attend to an unfamiliar adult with interest but show wariness or become anxious when that adult comes too close. (5–8 mos.; Parks 2004; Johnstone and Scherer 2000, 222) • Take the infant care teacher's hands and rock forward and backwards as a way of asking her to sing a favorite song. (8 mos.; Gustafson, Green, and West 1979; Kaye and Fogel 1980) • Engage in games such as pat-a-cake and peek-a-boo. (7–9 mos.; Coplan 1993, 3) • Make eye contact with a family member. • Vocalize to get an infant care teacher's attention.	• Move close to the infant care teacher and hold his hand when a visitor enters the classroom but watch the visitor with interest. (18 mos.; Meisels and others 2003) • Bring a familiar object to an adult when asked. (15–18 mos.; Parks 2004) • Allow an unfamiliar adult to get close only after the adult uses an object to bridge the interaction, such as showing interest in a toy that is also interesting to the child. (18 mos.; Meisels and others 2003) • Watch, and then help the infant care teacher as she prepares snack. • Seek reassurance from the infant care teacher when unsure if something is safe. (10–12 mos.; Fogel 2001, 305; Dickstein and Parke 1988; Hirshberg and Svejda 1990)	• Participate in storytelling with the infant care teacher. (30–36 mos.; Parks 2004) • Tell a teacher from the classroom next door about an upcoming birthday party. (36 mos.; Parks 2004) • Help the infant care teacher bring in the wheeled toys from the play yard at the end of the day. • Ask a classroom visitor her name.

Interactions with Adults

Behaviors leading up to the foundation (4 to 7 months)	Behaviors leading up to the foundation (9 to 17 months)	Behaviors leading up to the foundation (19 to 35 months)
During this period, the child may: • Engage in playful, face-to-face interactions with an adult, such as taking turns vocalizing and then smiling or laughing. (2–7 mos.; Lamb, Bornstein, and Teti 2002, 375) • Begin to protest separations from significant adults.	During this period, the child may: • Engage in back-and-forth interaction by handing a parent an object, then reaching to receive the object when it is handed back. (9–12 mos.; Lerner and Ciervo 2003) • Show—but not give—a toy to the infant care teacher. (9–12 mos.; Parks 2004)	During this period, the child may: • Practice being a grown-up during pretend play by dressing up or using a play stove. (18–36 mos.; Lerner and Dombro 2000) • Help the infant care teacher clean up after snack by putting snack dishes in the dish bin.

Foundation: Relationships with Adults

The development of close relationships with certain adults who provide consistent nurturance

8 months	*18 months*	*36 months*
At around eight months of age, children seek a special relationship with one (or a few) familiar adult(s) by initiating interactions and seeking proximity, especially when distressed. (6–9 mos.; Marvin and Britner 1999, 52)	At around 18 months of age, children feel secure exploring the environment in the presence of important adults with whom they have developed a relationship over an extended period of time. When distressed, children seek to be physically close to these adults. (6–18 mos.; Marvin and Britner 1999, 52; Bowlby 1983)	At around 36 months of age, when exploring the environment, from time to time children reconnect, in a variety of ways, with the adult(s) with whom they have developed a special relationship: through eye contact; facial expressions; shared feelings; or conversations about feelings, shared activities, or plans. When distressed, children may still seek to be physically close to these adults. (By 36 mos.; Marvin and Britner 1999, 57)
For example, the child may:	**For example, the child may:**	**For example, the child may:**
• Seek comfort from the infant care teacher by crying and looking for him. (7 mos.; Lamb, Bornstein, and Teti 2002, 372) • Cry out or follow after a parent when dropped off at the child care program. (6–9 mos.; Ainsworth1967, 4) • Lift her arms to be picked up by the special infant care teacher. (8 mos.; Meisels and others 2003, 17; Ainsworth 1967, 5) • Crawl toward a parent when startled by a loud noise. (8.5 mos.; Marvin and Britner 1999, 52) • Turn excitedly and raise his arms to greet a family member at pick-up time. (8 mos.; Ainsworth 1967, 5)	• Run in wide circles around the outdoor play area, circling back each time and hug the legs of the infant care teacher before running off again. • Snuggle with the special infant care teacher when feeling tired or grumpy. • Wave at the special infant care teacher from the top of the slide to make sure he is watching. • Follow a parent physically around the room. • Play away from the infant care teacher and then move close to him from time to time to check in. (12 mos.; Davies 2004, 10)	• Feel comfortable playing on the other side of the play yard away from the infant care teacher, but cry to be picked up after falling down. (24–36 mos.; Lamb, Bornstein, and Teti 2002, 376) • Call "Mama!" from across the room while playing with dolls to make sure that the mother is paying attention. (24–36 mos.; Schaffer and Emerson 1964) • Call for a family member and look out the window for him after being dropped off at school. (24–36 mos.; Marvin and Britner 1999, 56) • Communicate, "This is our favorite part" when reading a funny story with the infant care teacher. • Bring the grandmother's favorite book to her and express, "One more?" to see if she will read one more book, even though she has just said, "We're all done reading. Now it's time for nap." (Teti 1999; 18–36 mos.; Marvin and Britner 1999, 59) • Cry and look for the special infant care teacher after falling. • Seek the attention of the special infant care teacher and communicate, "Watch me!" before proudly displaying a new skill.

Relationships with Adults

Behaviors leading up to the foundation (4 to 7 months)	Behaviors leading up to the foundation (9 to 17 months)	Behaviors leading up to the foundation (19 to 35 months)
During this period, the child may: • Hold on to a parent's sweater when being held. (5 mos.; Marvin and Britner 1999, 51; Ainsworth 1967, 1) • Babble back and forth with the infant care teacher. (3–6 mos.; Caufield 1995) • Be more likely to smile when approached by the infant care teacher than a stranger. (3–6 mos.; Marvin and Britner 1999, 50) • Cry when an unfamiliar adult gets too close. (7 mos.; Bronson 1972)	During this period, the child may: • Cry and ask for a parent after being dropped off in the morning. (9–12 mos.; Lerner and Ciervo 2003) • Look for a smile from the infant care teacher when unsure if something is safe. (10–12 mos.; Fogel 2001, 305; Dickstein and Parke 1988; Hirshberg and Svejda 1990) • Cling to a parent when feeling ill. (10–11 mos.; Marvin and Britner 1999, 52)	During this period, the child may: • Say, "I go to school. Mama goes to work," after being dropped off in the morning. • Gesture for one more hug as a parent is leaving for work.

Foundation: Interactions with Peers

The developing ability to respond to and engage with other children

8 months	*18 months*	*36 months*
At around eight months of age, children show interest in familiar and unfamiliar peers. Children may stare at another child, explore another child's face and body, and respond to siblings and older peers. (8 mos.; Meisels and others 2003)	At around 18 months of age, children engage in simple back-and-forth interactions with peers for short periods of time. (Meisels and others 2003, 35)	At around 36 months of age, children engage in simple cooperative play with peers. (36 mos.; Meisels and others 2003 70)
For example, the child may:	**For example, the child may:**	**For example, the child may:**
• Watch other children with interest. (8 mos.; Meisels and others 2003) • Touch the eyes or hair of a peer. (8 mos.; Meisels and others 2003) • Attend to a crying peer with a serious expression. (7 mos.; American Academy of Pediatrics 2004, 212) • Laugh when an older sibling or peer makes a funny face. (8 mos.; Meisels and others 2003)	• Hit another child who takes a toy. (18 mos.; Meisels and others 2003, 35) • Offer a book to another child, perhaps with encouragement from the infant care teacher. (18 mos.; Meisels and others 2003, 35) • Tickle another child, get tickled back, and tickle him again. (18 mos.; Meisels and others 2003, 35) • Engage in reciprocal play, such as run-and-chase or offer-and-receive. (12–13 mos.; Howes 1988, v; 10–12 mos.; Ross and Goldman 1977) • Play ball with a peer by rolling the ball back and forth to each other. (12–15 mos.; Parks 2004; 9–16 mos.; Frankenburg and others 1990)	• Communicate with peers while digging in the sandbox together. (29–36 mos.; Hart and Risley 1999, 124) • Act out different roles with peers, sometimes switching in and out of her role. (By 36 mos.; Segal 2004, 44) • Build a tall tower with one or two other children. (36 mos.; Meisels and others 2003, 70) • Hand a peer a block or piece of railroad track when building.

Interactions with Peers

Behaviors leading up to the foundation (4 to 7 months)	Behaviors leading up to the foundation (9 to 17 months)	Behaviors leading up to the foundation (19 to 35 months)
During this period, the child may: • Notice other infants and children while sitting on a parent's or infant care teacher's lap. • Cry when hearing another baby cry. (4 mos.; Meisels and others 2003, 10)	During this period, the child may: • Engage in solitary play. (toddler; Segal 2004, 38) • Play a reciprocal game, such as pat-a-cake, with the infant care teacher and a peer. (7–11 mos.; Frankenburg and othres 1990)	During this period, the child may: • Use gestures to communicate a desire to play with a peer. (18–24 mos.; Parks 2004, 123) • Refuse to let a peer have a turn on the swing. (24 mos.; Meisels and others 2003, 45) • Push or bite when another child takes a toy. (24–30 mos.; Parks 2004) • Engage in complementary interactions, such as feeding a stuffed animal that another child is holding or pulling a friend in the wagon. (24–30 mos.; Meisels and others 2003, 57; Howes and Matheson 1992, 967) • Join a group of children who are together in one play space and follow them as they move outside. (30 mos.; Meisels and others 2003, 57)

Foundation: Relationships with Peers

The development of relationships with certain peers through interactions over time

8 months	*18 months*	*36 months*
At around eight months of age, children show interest in familiar and unfamiliar children. (8 mos.; Meisels and others 2003, 17)	At around 18 months of age, children prefer to interact with one or two familiar children in the group and usually engage in the same kind of back-and-forth play when interacting with those children. (12–18 mos.; Mueller and Lucas 1975)	At around 36 months of age, children have developed friendships with a small number of children in the group and engage in more complex play with those friends than with other peers.
For example, the child may:	**For example, the child may:**	**For example, the child may:**
• Watch other children with interest. (8 mos.; Meisels and others 2003) • Touch the eyes or hair of a peer. (8 mos.; Meisels and others 2003) • Attend to a crying peer with a serious expression. (7 mos.; American Academy of Pediatrics 2004, 212) • Laugh when an older sibling or peer makes a funny face. (8 mos.; Meisels and others 2003) • Try to get the attention of another child by smiling at him or babbling to him (6–9 mos.; Hay, Pederson, and Nash 1982)	• Play the same kind of game, such as run-and-chase, with the same peer almost every day. (Howes 1987, 259) • Choose to play in the same area as a friend. (Howes 1987, 259)	• Choose to play with a sibling instead of a less familiar child. (24–36 mos.; Dunn 1983, 795) • Exhibit sadness when the favorite friend is not at school one day. (24–36 mos.; Melson and Cohen 1981) • Seek one friend for running games and another for building with blocks. (Howes 1987) • Play "train" with one or two friends for an extended period of time by pretending that one is driving the train and the rest are riding.
Behaviors leading up to the foundation (4 to 7 months)	**Behaviors leading up to the foundation (9 to 17 months)**	**Behaviors leading up to the foundation (19 to 35 months)**
During this period, the child may: • Look at another child who is lying on the blanket nearby. (4 mos.; Meisels and others 2003, 10) • Turn toward the voice of a parent or older sibling. (4 mos.; Meisels and others 2003, 10)	During this period, the child may: • Watch an older sibling play nearby. (12 mos.; Meisels and others 2003, 26) • Bang blocks together next to a child who is doing the same thing. (12 mos.; Meisels and others 2003, 26) • Imitate the simple actions of a peer. (9–12 mos.; Ryalls, Gul, and Ryalls 2000)	During this period, the child may: • Engage in social pretend play with one or two friends; for example, pretend to be a dog while a friend pretends to be the owner. (24–30 mos.; Howes 1987, 261) • Express an interest in playing with a particular child. (13–24 mos.; Howes 1988, 3)

Foundation: Identity of Self in Relation to Others

The developing concept that the child is an individual operating within social relationships

8 months	*18 months*	*36 months*
At around eight months of age, children show clear awareness of being a separate person and of being connected with other people. Children identify others as both distinct from and connected to themselves. (Fogel 2001, 347)	At around 18 months of age, children demonstrate awareness of their characteristics and express themselves as distinct persons with thoughts and feelings. Children also demonstrate expectations of others' behaviors, responses, and characteristics on the basis of previous experiences with them.	At around 36 months of age, children identify their feelings, needs, and interests, and identify themselves and others as members of one or more groups by referring to categories. (24–36 mos.; Fogel 2001, 415; 18–30 mos.)
For example, the child may:	**For example, the child may:**	**For example, the child may:**
• Respond to someone who calls her name. (5–7 mos.; Parks 2004, 94; 9 mo.; Coplan 1993, 2) • Turn toward a familiar person upon hearing his name. (6–8 mos.; Parks 2004, 94; 8 mos.; Meisels and others 2003, 18) • Look at an unfamiliar adult with interest but show wariness or become anxious when that adult comes too close. (5–8 mos.; Parks 2004; Johnstone and Scherer 2000, 222) • Wave arms and kick legs when a parent enters the room. • Cry when the favorite infant care teacher leaves the room. (6–10 mos.; Parks 2004)	• Point to or indicate parts of the body when asked. (15–19 mos.; Parks 2004) • Express thoughts and feelings by saying "no!" (18 mos.; Meisels and others 2003) • Move excitedly when approached by an infant care teacher who usually engages in active play.	• Use pronouns such as I, me, you, we, he, and she. (By 36 mo.; American Academy of Pediatrics 2004, p. 307) • Say own name. (30–33 mos.; Parks 2004, 115) • Begin to make comparisons between self and others; for example, communicate, "_____ is a boy/girl like me." • Name people in the family. • Point to pictures of friends and say their names. • Communicate, "Do it myself!" when the infant care teacher tries to help.

Chart continues on next page.

Identity of Self in Relation to Others

Behaviors leading up to the foundation (4 to 7 months)	Behaviors leading up to the foundation (9 to 17 months)	Behaviors leading up to the foundation (19 to 35 months)
During this period, the child may: • Use hands to explore different parts of the body. (4 mos.; Kravitz, Goldenberg, and Neyhus 1978) • Examine her own hands and a parent's hands. (Scaled score of 9 for 4:06–4:15 mos.;* Bayley 2006, 53) • Watch or listen for the infant care teacher to come to meet the child's needs. (Birth–8 mos.; Lerner and Dombro 2000, 42)	During this period, the child may: • Play games such as peek-a-boo or run-and-chase with the infant care teacher. (Stern 1985, 102; 7–11 mos.; Frankenburg and others 1990) • Recognize familiar people, such as a neighbor or infant care teacher from another room, in addition to immediate family members. (12–18 mo.; Parks 2004) • Use names to refer to significant people; for example, "Mama" to refer to the mother and "Papa" to refer to the father. (11–14 mos.; Parks 2004, 109)	During this period, the child may: • Recognize his own image in the mirror and understand that it is himself. (Siegel 1999, 35; Lewis and Brooks-Gunn 1979, 56) • Know the names of familiar people, such as a neighbor. (by end of second year; American Academy of Pediatrics 2004, 270) • Show understanding of or use words such as you, me, mine, he, she, it, and I. (20–24 mos.; Parks 2004, 96; 20 mos.; Bayley 2006; 18–24 mos.; Lerner and Ciervo 2003; 19 mos.; Hart and Risley 1999, 61; 24–20 mos.; Parks 2004, 113) • Use name or other family label (e.g., nickname, birth order, "little sister") when referring to self. (18–24 mo.; Parks 2004; 24 mo.; Lewis and Brooks-Gunn 1979) • Claim everything as "mine." (24 mos.; Levine 1983) • Point to or indicate self in a photograph. (24 mos.; Lewis and Brooks-Gunn 1979) • Proudly show the infant care teacher a new possession. (24–30 mos.; Parks 2004)

*Four months, six days, to four months, 15 days.

Foundation: Recognition of Ability

The developing understanding that the child can take action to influence the environment

8 months	*18 months*	*36 months*
At around eight months of age, children understand that they are able to make things happen.	At around 18 months of age, children experiment with different ways of making things happen, persist in trying to do things even when faced with difficulty, and show a sense of satisfaction with what they can do. (McCarty, Clifton, and Collard 1999)	At around 36 months of age, children show an understanding of their own abilities and may refer to those abilities when describing themselves.
For example, the child may:	**For example, the child may:**	**For example, the child may:**
• Pat a musical toy to try to make the music come on again. (5–9 mos.; Parks 2004) • Raise arms to be picked up by the infant care teacher. (6–9 mos.; Fogel 2001, 274) • Initiate a favorite game; for example, hold out a foot to a parent to start a game of "This Little Piggy." (8 mos.; Meisels and others 2003; 6–9 mos.; Fogel 2001, 274) • Gesture at a book and smile with satisfaction after the infant care teacher gets it down from the shelf. (8 mos.; Meisels and others 2003)	• Roll a toy car back and forth on the ground and then push it really hard and let go to see what happens. (18 mos.; McCarty, Clifton, and Collard 1999) • Clap and bounce with joy after making a handprint with paint. (12–18 mos.; Sroufe 1979; Lally and others 1995, 71) • Squeeze a toy in different ways to hear the sounds it makes. (Scaled score of 10 for 13:16–14:15 mos.;* Bayley 2006) • Smile after walking up a steep incline without falling or carrying a bucket full of sand from one place to another without spilling. • Proudly hold up a book hidden in a stack after being asked by the infant care teacher to find it.	• Communicate, "I take care of the bunny" after helping to feed the class rabbit. (18–36 mos.; Lally and others 1995, 71) • Finish painting a picture and hold it up to show a family member. • Complete a difficult puzzle for the first time and clap or express, "I'm good at puzzles."

*Denotes thirteen months, 16 days, to fourteen months, 15 days.

Chart continues on next page.

Recognition of Ability

Behaviors leading up to the foundation (4 to 7 months)	Behaviors leading up to the foundation (9 to 17 months)	Behaviors leading up to the foundation (19 to 35 months)
During this period, the child may: • Try again and again to roll over, even though not yet able to roll completely over. • Grasp, suck, or look at a teething ring. (Before 8 mos. of age; Fogel 2001, 218) • Shake a toy, hear it make noise, and shake it again. • Stop crying upon seeing the infant care teacher approach with a bottle.	During this period, the child may: • Drop a blanket over the side of the crib and wait for the infant care teacher to pick it up. (12 mos.; Meisels and others 2003) • Drop a toy truck in the water table and blink in anticipation of the big splash. (12 mos.; Meisels and others 2003) • Look over a shoulder, smile at the mother, and giggle in a playful way while crawling past her, to entice her to play a game of run-and-chase. (10–14 mos.; Bayley 2006) • Turn light switch on and off repeatedly.	During this period, the child may: • Insist on zipping up a jacket when the infant care teacher tries to help. (20–28 mos.; Hart and Risley 1999, 62; 24 mos.; Hart and Risley 1999, 122 and 129; 20–36 mos.; Bates 1990; Bullock and Lutkenhaus 1988, 1990; Stipek, Gralinski, and Kopp 1990) • Point to a stack of blocks he has made and express, "look" to the infant care teacher. (28 mos.; Hart and Risley 1999, 96) • Communicate, "I doing this," "I don't do this, " "I can do this," or "I did this." (25 mos.; Hart and Risley 1999, 121; Dunn, 1987; Stipek, Gralinski, and Kopp 1990) • Say, "I climb high" when telling the infant care teacher about what happened during outside play time, then run outside to show him how. (30 mos.; Meisels and others 2003)

Foundation: Expression of Emotion

The developing ability to express a variety of feelings through facial expressions, movements, gestures, sounds, or words

8 months	*18 months*	*36 months*
At around eight months of age, children express a variety of primary emotions such as contentment, distress, joy, sadness, interest, surprise, disgust, anger, and fear. (Lamb, Bornstein, and Teti 2002, 341)	At around 18 months of age, children express emotions in a clear and intentional way, and begin to express some complex emotions, such as pride.	At around 36 months of age, children express complex, self-conscious emotions such as pride, embarrassment, shame, and guilt. Children demonstrate awareness of their feelings by using words to describe feelings to others or acting them out in pretend play. (Lewis and others 1989; Lewis 2000b; Lagattuta and Thompson 2007)
For example, the child may:	**For example, the child may:**	**For example, the child may:**
• Exhibit wariness, cry, or turn away when a stranger approaches. (6 mos.; Lamb, Bornstein, and Teti 2002, 338; Fogel 2001, 297; 7–8 mos.; Lewis 2000a, 277) • Be more likely to react with anger than just distress when accidentally hurt by another child. (later in the first year; Lamb, Bornstein, and Teti 2002, 341) • Express fear of unfamiliar people by moving near a familiar infant care teacher. (8 mos.; Bronson 1972) • Stop crying and snuggle after being picked up by a parent. • Show surprise when the infant care teacher removes the blanket covering her face to start a game of peek-a-boo.	• Show affection for a family member by hugging. (8–18 mos.; Lally and others 1995; Greenspan and Greenspan 1985, 84) • Express jealousy by trying to crowd onto the infant care teacher's lap when another child is already sitting there. (12–18 mos.; Hart and others 1998) • Express anger at having a toy taken away by taking it back out of the other child's hands or hitting her. (18 mos.; Squires, Bricker, and Twombly 2002, 115) • Smile directly at other children when interacting with them. (18 mos.; Squires, Bricker, and Twombly 2002, 115) • Express pride by communicating, "I did it!" (15–24 mos.; Lewis and others 1989; Lewis 2000b)	• Hide face with hands when feeling embarrassed. (Lagattuta and Thompson 2007) • Use words to describe feelings; for example, "I don't like that." (24–36 mos.; Fogel 2001, 414; 24–36 mos.; Harris and others 1989; Yuill 1984) • Communicate, "I miss Grandma," after talking on the phone with her. (24–36 mos.; Harris and others 1989; Yuill 1984) • Act out different emotions during pretend play by "crying" when pretending to be sad and "cooing" when pretending to be happy. (Dunn, Bretherton, and Munn 1987) • Express guilt after taking a toy out of another child's cubby without permission by trying to put it back without anyone seeing. (Lagattuta and Thompson 2007)

Chart continues on next page.

Expression of Emotion

Behaviors leading up to the foundation (4 to 7 months)	Behaviors leading up to the foundation (9 to 17 months)	Behaviors leading up to the foundation (19 to 35 months)
During this period, the child may: • Get frustrated or angry when unable to reach a toy. (4–6 mos.; Sternberg, Campos, and Emde 1983) • Express joy by squealing. (5–6 mos.; Parks 2004, 125) • Frown and make noises to indicate frustration. (5–6 mos.; Parks 2004, 125) • Be surprised when something unexpected happens. (First 6 mos. of life; Lewis 2000a)	During this period, the child may: • Become anxious when a parent leaves the room. (6–9 mos.; Parks 2004) • Knock a shape-sorter toy away when it gets to be too frustrating. (10–12 mos.; Sroufe 1979) • Show anger, when another child takes a toy, by taking it back. (10–12 mos.; Sroufe 1979) • Express fear by crying upon hearing a dog bark loudly or seeing someone dressed in a costume. (10 mos.; Bronson 1972) • Express sadness by frowning after losing or misplacing a favorite toy. (9–10 mos.; Fogel 2001, 300) • Smile with affection as a sibling approaches. (10 mos.; Sroufe 1979; Fox and Davidson 1988) • Push an unwanted object away. (12 mos.; Squires, Bricker, and Twombly 2002, 114)	During this period, the child may: • Communicate, "Mama mad" after being told by the mother to stop an action. (28 mos.; Bretherton and others 1986) • Use one or a few words to describe feelings to the infant care teacher. (18–30 mos.; Bretherton and others 1986; Dunn 1987) • Express frustration through tantrums. (18–36 mos.; Pruett 1999, 148)

Foundation: Empathy

The developing ability to share in the emotional experiences of others

8 months	*18 months*	*36 months*
At around eight months of age, children demonstrate awareness of others' feelings by reacting to their emotional expressions.	At around 18 months of age, children change their behavior in response to the feelings of others even though their actions may not always make the other person feel better. Children show an increased understanding of the reason for another's distress and may become distressed by the other's distress. (14 mos.; Zahn-Waxler, Robinson, and Emde 1992; Thompson 1987; 24 mos.; Zahn-Waxler and Radke-Yarrow 1982, 1990)	At around 36 months of age, children understand that other people have feelings that are different from their own and can sometimes respond to another's distress in a way that might make that person feel better. (24–36 mos.; Hoffman 1982; 18 mos.; Thompson 1987, 135).
For example, the child may:	**For example, the child may:**	**For example, the child may:**
• Stop playing and look at a child who is crying. (7 mos.; American Academy of Pediatrics 2004, 212) • Laugh when an older sibling or peer makes a funny face. (8 mos.; Meisels and others 2003) • Return the smile of the infant care teacher. • Grimace when another child cries. (Older than 6 mos.; Wingert and Brant 2005, 35)	• Offer to help a crying playmate by bringing his own mother over. (13–15 mos.; Wingert and Brant 2005, 35) • Try to hug a crying peer. (18 mos.; Thompson 1987, 135) • Bring her own special blanket to a peer who is crying. (13–15 mos.; Wingert and Brant 2005, 35) • Become upset when another child throws a tantrum. • Gently pat a crying peer on his back, just like his infant care teacher did earlier in the day. (16 mos.; Bergman and Wilson 1984; Zahn-Waxler and others 1992) • Hit a child who is crying loudly. • Stop playing and look with concerned attention at a child who is screaming. • Move quickly away from a child who is crying loudly.	• Do a silly dance in an attempt to make a crying peer smile. (24–36 mos.; Dunn 1988) • Communicate, "Lucas is sad because Isabel took his cup." (36 mos.; Harris and others 1989; Yuill 1984) • Comfort a younger sibling who is crying by patting his back, expressing "It's okay" and offering him a snack. (Denham 1998, 34) • Communicate, "Mama sad" when the mother cries during a movie. (24–36 mos.; Dunn 1994; Harris 2000, 282). • Communicate, "Olivia's mama is happy" and point to or indicate the illustration in the picture book. (24 mos.; Harris 2000, 282). • Get an infant care teacher to help a child who has fallen down and is crying.

Chart continues on next page.

Empathy

Behaviors leading up to the foundation (4 to 7 months)	Behaviors leading up to the foundation (9 to 17 months)	Behaviors leading up to the foundation (19 to 35 months)
During this period, the child may: • Cry when hearing another baby cry. (Younger than 6 mos; Wingert and Brant 2005, 35)	During this period, the child may: • Stand nearby and quietly watch a peer who has fallen down and is crying. • Exhibit social referencing by looking for emotional indicators in others' faces, voices, or gestures to decide what to do when uncertain. (10–12 mos.; Thompson 1987, 129) • Cry upon hearing another child cry. (12 mos.; Meisels and others 2003, 26)	During this period, the child may: • Hug a crying peer. (18–24 mos.; Parks 2004, 123) • Become upset in the presence of those who are upset.

Foundation: Emotion Regulation

The developing ability to manage emotional responses, with assistance from others and independently

8 months	*18 months*	*36 months*
At around eight months of age, children use simple behaviors to comfort themselves and begin to communicate the need for help to alleviate discomfort or distress.	At around 18 months of age, children demonstrate a variety of responses to comfort themselves and actively avoid or ignore situations that cause discomfort. Children can also communicate needs and wants through the use of a few words and gestures. (National Research Council and Institute of Medicine 2000, 112; 15–18 mos.; American Academy of Pediatrics 2004, 270; Coplan 1993, 1)	At around 36 months of age, children anticipate the need for comfort and try to prepare themselves for changes in routine. Children have many self-comforting behaviors to choose from, depending on the situation, and can communicate specific needs and wants. (Kopp 1989; CDE 2005)
For example, the child may:	**For example, the child may:**	**For example, the child may:**
• Turn away from an overstimulating activity. (3–12 mos.; Rothbart, Ziaie, and O'Boyle 1992) • Vocalize to get a parent's attention. (6.5–8 mos.; Parks 2004, 126) • Lift arms to the infant care teacher to communicate a desire to be held. (7–9 mos.; Coplan 1993, 3; 5–9 mos.; Parks 2004, 121) • Turn toward the infant care teacher for assistance when crying. (6–9 mos.; Fogel 2001, 274) • Cry after her hand was accidentally stepped on by a peer and then hold the hand up to the infant care teacher to look at it. • Reach toward a bottle that is up on the counter and vocalize when hungry. • Make a face of disgust to tell the infant care teacher that he does not want any more food. (6–9 mos.; Lerner and Ciervo 2003) • Bump head, cry, and look to infant care teacher for comfort. • Suck on a thumb to make self feel better. • Look at the infant care teacher when an unfamiliar person enters the room.	• Use gestures and simple words to express distress and seek specific kinds of assistance from the infant care teacher in order to calm self. (Brazelton 1992; Kopp 1989, 347) • Use comfort objects, such as a special blanket or stuffed toy, to help calm down. (Kopp 1989, 348) • Seek to be close to a parent when upset. (Lieberman 1993) • Play with a toy as a way to distract self from discomfort. (12–18 mos.; Kopp 1989, 347) • Communicate, "I'm okay" after falling down. (National Research Council and Institute of Medicine 2000, 112) • Indicate her knee and say "boo boo" after falling down and gesture or ask for a bandage. • Approach the infant care teacher for a hug and express, "Mommy work," then point to the door to communicate missing the mother.	• Reach for the mother's hand just before she pulls a bandage off the child's knee. • Ask the infant care teacher to hold him up to the window to wave good-bye before the parent leaves in the morning. • Show the substitute teacher that she likes a back rub during naptime by patting own back while lying on the mat. • Play quietly in a corner of the room right after drop-off, until ready to play with the other children. • Ask the infant care teacher to explain what's going to happen at the child's dental appointment later in the day. • Communicate, "Daddy always comes back" after saying good-bye to him in the morning.

Chart continues on next page.

Emotion Regulation

Behaviors leading up to the foundation (4 to 7 months)	Behaviors leading up to the foundation (9 to 17 months)	Behaviors leading up to the foundation (19 to 35 months)
During this period, the child may: • Suck on hands, focus on an interesting toy, or move the body in a rocking motion to calm self. (3–6 mos.; Parks 2004, 10) • Cry inconsolably less often than in the early months. (6 mos.; Parks 2004, 10) • Calm self by sucking on fingers or hands. (4 mos.; Thelen and Fogel 1989; 3–12 mos.; Bronson 2000b, 64) • Be able to inhibit some negative emotions. (Later in the first year; Fox and Calkins 2000) • Shift attention away from a distressing event onto an object, as a way of managing emotions. (6 mos.; Weinberg and others 1999) • Fall asleep when feeling overwhelmed.	During this period, the child may: • Move away from something that is bothersome and move toward the infant care teacher for comfort. (6–12 mos.; Bronson 2000b, 64) • Fight back tears when a parent leaves for the day. (12 mos.; Bridges, Grolnick, and Connell 1997; Parritz 1996; Sroufe 1979) • Look for a cue from the infant care teacher when unsure if something is safe. (10–12 mos.; Fogel 2001, 305; Dickstein and Parke 1988; Hirshberg and Svejda 1990) • Fuss to communicate needs or wants; begin to cry if the infant care teacher does not respond soon enough. (11–19 mos.; Hart and Risley 1999, 77) • Repeat sounds to get the infant care teacher's attention. (11–19 mos.; Hart and Risley 1999, 79)	During this period, the child may: • Continue to rely on adults for reassurance and help in controlling feelings and behavior. (Lally and others 1995) • Reenact emotional events in play to try to gain mastery over these feelings. (Greenspan and Greenspan 1985) • Use words to ask for specific help with regulating emotions. (Kopp 1989) • Express wants and needs verbally; for example, say, "hold me" to the infant care teacher when feeling tired or overwhelmed. (30–31.5 mos.; Parks 2004, 130)

Foundation: Impulse Control

The developing capacity to wait for needs to be met, to inhibit potentially hurtful behavior, and to act according to social expectations, including safety rules

8 months	*18 months*	*36 months*
At around eight months of age, children act on impulses. (Birth–9 mos.; Bronson 2000b, 64)	At around 18 months of age, children respond positively to choices and limits set by an adult to help control their behavior. (18 mos.; Meisels and others 2003, 34; Kaler and Kopp 1990)	At around 36 months of age, children may sometimes exercise voluntary control over actions and emotional expressions. (Bronson 2000b, 67)
For example, the child may:	**For example, the child may:**	**For example, the child may:**
• Explore the feel of hair by pulling it. (4–7 mos.; American Academy of Pediatrics 2004, 226) • Reach for an interesting toy that another child is mouthing. • Reach for another child's bottle that was just set down nearby. • Turn the head away or push the bottle away when finished eating (8 mos.; Meisels and others 2003, 19).	• Stop drawing on the wall when a parent asks. (18 mos.; Meisels and others 2003) • Choose one toy when the infant care teacher asks, "Which one do you want?" even though the child really wants both. • Express "no no" while approaching something the child knows she should not touch, because the infant care teacher has communicated "no no" in the past when the child tried to do this. • Look to the infant care teacher to see his reaction when the child reaches toward the light switch. • Stop reaching for the eyeglasses on the infant care teacher's face when she gently says, "no no." (Scaled score of 10 for 7:16–8:15 mos.; Bayley 2006, 87; 12 mos.; Meisels and others 2003, 27)	• Jump up and down on the couch but stop jumping and climb down when a parent enters the room. (36 mos.; Meisels and others 2003) • Experience difficulty (e.g., cry, whine, pout) with transitions. (30–36 mos.; Parks 2004, 320) • Begin to share. • Handle transitions better when prepared ahead of time or when the child has some control over what happens. • Touch a pet gently without needing to be reminded. • Wait to start eating until others at the table are also ready.

Chart continues on next page.

Impulse Control

Behaviors leading up to the foundation (4 to 7 months)	Behaviors leading up to the foundation (9 to 17 months)	Behaviors leading up to the foundation (19 to 35 months)
During this period, the child may: • Cry when hungry or tired. • Fall asleep when tired.	During this period, the child may: • Crawl too close to a younger infant lying nearby. • Refrain from exploring another baby's hair when reminded to be gentle. (8–10 mos.; Brazelton 1992, 256) • Look at the infant care teacher's face to determine whether it is all right to play with a toy on the table. (12 mos.; Meisels and others 2003, 25) • Bite another child who takes a toy. • Reach for food on a plate before the infant care teacher offers it. (12 mos.; Meisels and others 2003, 25)	During this period, the child may: • Begin to use words and dramatic play to describe, understand, and control impulses and feelings. (Lally and others 1995) • Communicate, "Mine!" and take a doll out of the hands of a peer. (23–24 mos.; Parks 2004, 330) • Throw a puzzle piece on the floor after having trouble fitting it in the opening. (24 mos.; Meisels and others 2003) • Open the playground door and run out, even after being asked by the infant care teacher to wait. (24 mos.; Meisels and others 2003) • Start to take another child's toy, then stop after catching the eye of the infant care teacher. (24 mos.; Meisels and others 2003) • Use a quiet voice at naptime. (30 mos.; Meisels and others 2003) • Understand and carry out simple commands or rules. (Bronson 2000b, 85) • Have a tantrum rather than attempt to manage strong feelings. (Brazelton 1992) • Be able to wait for a turn.

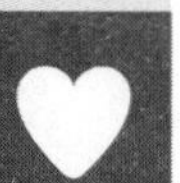

Foundation: Social Understanding

The developing understanding of the responses, communication, emotional expressions, and actions of other people

8 months	*18 months*	*36 months*
At around eight months of age, children have learned what to expect from familiar people, understand what to do to get another's attention, engage in back-and-forth interactions with others, and imitate the simple actions or facial expressions of others.	At around 18 months of age, children know how to get the infant care teacher to respond in a specific way through gestures, vocalizations, and shared attention; use another's emotional expressions to guide their own responses to unfamiliar events; and learn more complex behavior through imitation. Children also engage in more complex social interactions and have developed expectations for a greater number of familiar people.	At around 36 months of age, children can talk about their own wants and feelings and those of other people, describe familiar routines, participate in coordinated episodes of pretend play with peers, and interact with adults in more complex ways.
For example, the child may:	**For example, the child may:**	**For example, the child may:**
• Smile when the infant care teacher pauses, to get her to continue playing peek-a-boo or pat-a-cake. • Squeal in anticipation of the infant care teacher's uncovering her eyes during a game of peek-a-boo. • Learn simple behaviors by imitating a parent's facial expressions, gestures, or sounds. • Try to get a familiar game or routine started by prompting the infant care teacher. • Quiet crying upon realizing that the infant care teacher is approaching.	• Gesture toward a desired toy or food while reaching, making imperative vocal sounds, and looking toward the infant care teacher. • Seek reassurance from the infant care teacher when unsure about something. • Vary response to different infant care teachers depending on their play styles, even before they have started playing; for example, get very excited upon seeing an infant care teacher who regularly plays in an exciting, vigorous manner. • Engage in back-and-forth play that involves turn-taking, such as rolling a ball back and forth. • Look in the direction of the infant care teacher's gesturing or pointing. • Learn more complex behaviors through imitation, such as watching an older child put toys together and then doing it.	• Name own feelings or desires, explicitly contrast them with another's, or describe why the child feels the way he does. • Describe what happens during the bedtime routine or another familiar everyday event. • Move into and out of pretend play roles, tell other children what they should do in their roles, or extend the sequence (such as by asking "Wanna drink?" after bringing a pretend hamburger to the table as a waiter). • Help the infant care teacher search for a missing toy. • Talk about what happened during a recent past experience, with the assistance of the infant care teacher. • Help the infant care teacher clean up at the end of the day by putting the toys in the usual places.

Chart continues on next page.

Social Understanding

Behaviors leading up to the foundation (4 to 7 months)	Behaviors leading up to the foundation (9 to 17 months)	Behaviors leading up to the foundation (19 to 35 months)
During this period, the child may: • Make imperative vocal sounds to attract the infant care teacher's attention. • Participate in playful, face-to-face interactions with an adult, such as taking turns vocalizing.	During this period, the child may: • Follow the infant care teacher's gaze to look at a toy. • Hold up or gesture toward objects in order to direct the infant care teacher's attention to them.	During this period, the child may: • Vary play with different peers depending on their preferred play activities. • Imitate the behavior of peers as well as adults.

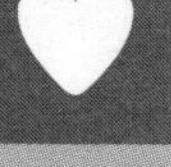

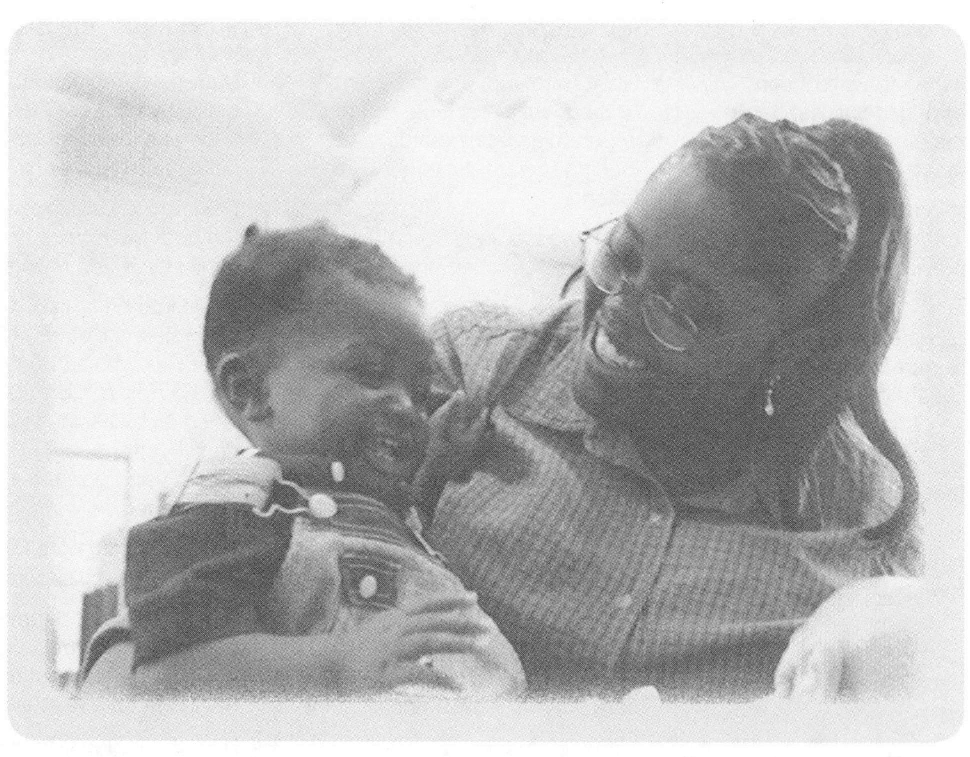

References

Ainsworth, M. D. 1967. *Infancy in Uganda: Infant Care and the Growth of Love.* Baltimore: Johns Hopkins University Press.

American Academy of Pediatrics. 2004. *Caring for Your Baby and Young Child: Birth to Age 5* (Fourth edition). Edited by S. P. Shelov and R. E. Hannemann. New York: Bantam Books.

Anderson, C., and D. Keltner. 2002. "The Role of Empathy in the Formation and Maintenance of Social Bonds," *Behavioral and Brain Sciences,* Vol. 25, No. 1, 21–22.

Barrera, M. E., and D. Maurer. 1981. "Discrimination of Strangers by the Three-Month-Old," *Child Development,* Vol. 52, No. 2, 558–63.

Barrett, L., and others. 2007. "The Experience of Emotion," *Annual Review of Psychology,* Vol. 58, 373–403.

Bates, E. 1990. "Language About Me and You: Pronomial Reference and the Emerging Concept of Self," in *The Self in Transition: Infancy to Childhood.* Edited by D. Cicchetti and M. Beeghly. Chicago: University of Chicago Press.

Bayley, N. 2006. *Bayley Scales of Infant and Toddler Development* (Third edition). San Antonio, TX: Harcourt Assessment, Inc.

Bell, M., and C. Wolfe. 2004. "Emotion and Cognition: An Intricately Bound Developmental Process," *Child Development,* Vol. 75, No. 2, 366–70.

Bergman, A., and A. Wilson. 1984. "Thoughts About Stages on the Way to Empathy and the Capacity for Concern," in *Empathy II.* Edited by J. Lichtenberg, M. Bornstein, and D. Silver. Hillsdale, NJ: Lawrence Erlbaum Associates.

Bowlby, J. 1983. *Attachment* (Second edition), Attachment and Loss series, Vol. 1. Foreword by Allan N. Schore. New York: Basic Books.

Brazelton, T. B. 1992. *Touchpoints: Your Child's Emotional and Behavioral Development.* New York: Perseus Publishing.

Bretherton, I., and others. 1986. "Learning to Talk About Emotions: A Functionalist Perspective," *Child Development,* Vol. 57, 529–48.

Bridges, L. J.; W. S. Grolnick; and J. P Connell. 1997. "Infant Emotion Regulation with Mothers and Fathers," *Infant Behavior and Development,* Vol. 20, 47–57.

Bronson, G. W. 1972. "Infants' Reaction to Unfamiliar Persons and Novel Objects," *Monographs of the Society for Research in Child Development,* Vol. 37, No. 148, 1–46.

Bronson, M. 2000a. "Recognizing and Supporting the Development of Self-Regulation in Young Children," *Young Children,* Vol. 55, No. 2, 32–37.

Bronson, M. 2000b. *Self-Regulation in Early Childhood: Nature and Nurture.* New York: Guilford Press.

Bullock, M., and P. Lutkenhaus. 1988. "The Development of Volitional Behavior in the Toddler Years," *Child Development,* Vol. 59, 664–74.

Bullock, M., and P. Lutkenhaus. 1990. "Who Am I? Self-Understanding in Toddlers," *Merrill-Palmer Quarterly,* Vol. 36, 217–38.

Burk, D. I. 1996. "Understanding Friendship and Social Interaction," *Childhood Education,* Vol. 72, No. 5, 282–85.

Cacioppo, J., and G. Berntson. 1999. "The Affect System: Architecture and Operating Characteristics," *Current Directions in Psychological Science,* Vol. 8, No. 5, 133–37.

California Department of Education (CDE). 2005. "Desired Results Developmental Profile (DRDP)." Sacramento: California Department of Education.

http://www.cde.ca.gov/sp/cd/ci/desiredresults.asp (accessed February 7, 2007).

Campos, J.; C. Frankel; and L. Camras. 2004. "On the Nature of Emotion Regulation," *Child Development,* Vol. 75, No. 2, 377–94.

Caufield, R. 1995. "Reciprocity Between Infants and Caregivers During the First Year of Life," *Early Childhood Education Journal,* Vol. 23, No. 1, 3–8.

Cheah, C., and K. Rubin. 2003. "European American and Mainland Chinese Mothers' Socialization Beliefs Regarding Preschoolers' Social Skills," *Parenting: Science and Practice,* Vol. 3, No. 1, 1–21

Cohen, J., and others. 2005. *Helping Young Children Succeed: Strategies to Promote Early Childhood Social and Emotional Development.* Washington, DC: National Conference of State Legislatures and Zero to Three. http://www.zerotothree.org/policy (accessed on December 7, 2006)

Connell, J. P. 1990. "Context, Self, and Action: A Motivational Analysis of Self-System Processes Across the Lifespan," in *The Self in Transition: Infancy to Childhood.* Edited by D. Cicchetti and M. Beeghly. Chicago: The University of Chicago Press.

Coplan, J. 1993. *Early Language Milestone Scale: Examiner's Manual* (Second edition). Austin, TX: Pro-ed.

Davies, D. 2004. *Child Development: A Practitioner's Guide* (Second edition). New York: Guilford Press.

DeCasper, A. J., and W. P. Fifer. 1980. "Of Human Bonding: Newborns Prefer Their Mothers' Voices," *Science,* Vol. 208, No. 6, 1174–76.

Denham, S. 1998. *Emotional Development in Young Children.* New York: Guilford Press.

Denham, S., and R. Weissberg. 2003. "Social-Emotional Learning in Early Childhood: What We Know and Where to Go From Here," in *A Blueprint for the Promotion of Prosocial Behavior in Early Childhood.* Edited by E. Chesebrough and others. New York: Kluwer Academic/Plenum Publishers.

Dickstein, S., and R. D. Parke. 1988. "Social Referencing in Infancy: A Glance at Fathers and Marriage," *Child Development,* Vol. 59, No. 2, 506–11.

Dunn, J. 1983. "Sibling Relationships in Early Childhood," *Child Development,* Vol. 54, No. 4, 787–811.

Dunn, J. 1987. "The Beginnings of Moral Understanding: Development in the Second Year," in *The Emergence of Morality in Young Children.* Edited by J. Kagan and S. Lamb. Chicago: University of Chicago Press.

Dunn, J. 1988. *The Beginnings of Social Understanding.* Cambridge, MA: Harvard University Press.

Dunn, J. 1994. "Changing Minds and Changing Relationships," in *Children's Early Understanding of Mind: Origins and Development.* Edited by C. Lewis and P. Mitchell. Hillsdale, NJ: Lawrence Erlbaum Associates.

Dunn, J.; I. Bretherton; and P. Munn. 1987. "Conversations About Feeling States Between Mothers and Their Young Children," *Developmental Psychology,* Vol. 23, No. 1, 132–39.

Eisenberg, N. 2000. "Emotion, Regulation and Moral Development," *Annual Review of Psychology,* Vol. 51, 665–97.

Eisenberg, N.; C. Champion; and Y. Ma. 2004. "Emotion-Related Regulation: An Emerging Construct," *Merrill-Palmer Quarterly,* Vol. 50, No. 3, 236–59.

Eisenberg, N., and others. 1993. "The Relations of Emotionality and Regulation to Preschoolers' Social Skills and Sociometric Status," *Child Development,* Vol. 64, 1418–38.

Eisenberg, N., and T. Spinrad. 2004. "Emotion-Related Regulation: Sharpening the Definition," *Child Development,* Vol. 75, No. 2, 334–39.

Fabes, R., and others. 2001. "Preschoolers' Spontaneous Emotion Vocabulary: Relations to Likability," *Early Education & Development,* Vol. 12, No. 1, 11–27.

Fernald, A. 1993. "Approval and Disapproval: Infant Responsiveness to Vocal Affect in Familiar and Unfamiliar Languages," *Child Development,* Vol. 64, No. 3, 657–74.

Fogel, A. 2001. *Infancy: Infant, Family, and Society* (Fourth edition). Belmont, CA: Wadsworth/Thomson Learning.

Fox, N. A., and S. D. Calkins. 2000. "Multiple Measure Approaches to the Study of Infant Emotion," in *Handbook of Emotions* (Second edition). Edited by M. Lewis and J. M. Haviland-Jones. New York: Guilford Press.

Fox, N. A., and R. J. Davidson. 1988. "Patterns of Brain Electrical Activity During the Expression of Discrete Emotions in Ten-Month-Old Infants," *Developmental Psychology,* Vol. 24, 230–36.

Frankenburg, W. K., and others. 1990. *Denver II Screening Manual.* Denver, CO: Denver Developmental Materials.

Fredrickson, B. 2000. "Cultivating Positive Emotions to Optimize Health and Well-Being," *Prevention and Treatment,* Vol. 3, No. 1.

Fredrickson, B. 2003. "The Value of Positive Emotions," *American Scientist,* Vol. 91, 330–35.

Greenspan, S., and N. T. Greenspan. 1985. *First Feelings: Milestones in the Emotional Development of Your Baby and Child.* New York: Penguin Books.

Gustafson, G. E.; J. A. Green; and M. J. West. 1979. "The Infant's Changing Role in Mother-Infant Games: The Growth of Social Skills," *Infant Behavior and Development,* Vol. 2, 301–8.

Harris, P. L. 2000. "Understanding Emotion," in *Handbook of Emotions* (Second edition). Edited by M. Lewis and J. M. Haviland-Jones. New York: Guilford Press.

Harris, P. L., and others. 1989. "Young Children's Theory of Mind and Emotion," *Cognition and Emotion,* Vol. 3, No. 4, 379–400.

Hart, B., and T. R. Risley. 1999. *The Social World of Children: Learning to Talk.* Baltimore, MD: Paul H. Brookes Publishing.

Hart, S., and others. 1998. "Jealousy Protests in Infants of Depressed Mothers," *Infant Behavior and Development,* Vol. 21, No. 1, 137–48.

Hay, D. F.; J. Pederson; and A. Nash. 1982. "Dyadic Interaction in the First Year of Life," in *Peer Relationships and Social Skills in Childhood.* Edited by K. H. Rubin and H. S. Ross. New York: Springer-Verlag.

Hirshberg, L. M., and M. Svejda. 1990. "When Infants Look to Their Parents: Infants' Social Referencing of Mothers Compared to Fathers," *Child Development,* Vol. 61, No. 4, 1175–86.

Hoffman, M. L. 1982. "Development of Prosocial Motivation: Empathy and Guilt," in *The Development of Prosocial Behavior.* Edited by N. Eisenberg. New York: Academic Press.

Howes, C. 1983. "Patterns of Friendship," *Child Development,* Vol. 54, No. 4, 1041–53.

Howes, C. 1987. "Social Competence with Peers in Young Children: Developmental Sequences," *Developmental Review,* Vol. 7, 252–72.

Howes, C. 1988. "Peer Interaction of Young Children," *Monographs of the Society for Research in Child Development,* Vol. 53, No. 1.

Howes, C., and C. C. Matheson. 1992. "Sequences in the Development of Competent Play with Peers: Social and Social Pretend Play," *Developmental Psychology,* Vol. 28, No. 5, 961–74.

Johnson, M., and others. 1991. "Newborns' Preferential Tracking of Face-Like Stimuli and Its Subsequent Decline," *Cognition,* Vol. 40, Nos. 1-2, 1–19.

Johnstone, T., and K. R., Scherer. 2000. "Vocal Communication of Emotion," in *Handbook of Emotions* (Second edition). Edited by M. Lewis and J. Haviland-Jones. New York: Guilford Press.

Kaler, S. R., and C. B. Kopp. 1990. "Compliance and Comprehension in Very Young Toddlers," *Child Development*, Vol. 61, No. 6, 1997–2003.

Kaye, K., and A. Fogel. 1980. "The Temporal Structure of Face-to-Face Communication Between Mothers and Infants," *Developmental Psychology*, Vol. 16, 454–64.

Kontos, S., and A. Wilcox-Herzog. January, 1997. "Research in Review: Teacher's Interactions with Children: Why Are They So Important?" *Young Children*, Vol. 52, No. 2, 4–12.

Kopp, C. 1989. "Regulation of Distress and Negative Emotions: A Developmental View," *Developmental Psychology*, Vol. 25, No. 3, 343–54.

Kravitz, H.; D. Goldenberg; and A. Neyhus. 1978. "Tactual Exploration by Normal Infants," *Developmental Medicine and Child-Neurology*, Vol. 20, No. 6, 720–26.

Lagattuta, K. H., and R. A. Thompson. 2007. "The Development of Self-Conscious Emotions: Cognitive Processes and Social Influences," in *The Self-Conscious Emotions: Theory and Research*. Edited by J. L. Tracy, R. W. Robins, and J. P. Tangney. New York: Guilford Press.

Lally, J. R., and others. 1995. *Caring for Infants and Toddlers in Groups: Developmentally Appropriate Practice*. Washington, DC: Zero to Three Press.

Lamb, M. E.; M. H. Bornstein; and D. M. Teti. 2002. *Development in Infancy: An Introduction* (Fourth edition). Mahwah, NJ: Lawrence Erlbaum Associates.

Lerner, C., and L. A. Ciervo. 2003. *Healthy Minds: Nurturing Children's Development from 0 to 36 Months*. Washington, DC: Zero to Three Press and American Academy of Pediatrics.

Lerner, C., and A. L. Dombro. 2000. *Learning and Growing Together: Understanding and Supporting Your Child's Development*. Washington, DC: Zero to Three Press.

Levenson, R., and A. Ruef. 1992. "Empathy: A Physiological Substrate," *Journal of Personality and Social Psychology*, Vol. 63, No. 2, 234–46.

Levine, L. E. 1983. "Mine: Self-Definition in 2-Year-Old Boys," *Developmental Psychology*, Vol. 19, 544–49.

Lewis, M. 2000a. "The Emergence of Human Emotions," in *Handbook of Emotions* (Second edition). Edited by M. Lewis and J. M. Haviland-Jones. New York: Guilford Press.

Lewis, M. 2000b. "Self-Conscious Emotions: Embarrassment, Pride, Shame, and Guilt," in *Handbook of Emotions* (Second edition). Edited by M. Lewis and J. M. Haviland-Jones. New York: Guilford Press.

Lewis, M., and J. Brooks-Gunn. 1979. *Social Cognition and the Acquisition of Self*. New York: Plenum Press.

Lewis, M., and others. 1989. "Self Development and Self-Conscious Emotions," *Child Development*, Vol. 60, No. 1, 146–56.

Lieberman, A. F. 1993. *The Emotional Life of the Toddler*. New York: Free Press.

Marvin, R., and P. Britner. 1999. "Normative Development: The Ontogeny of Attachment," in *Handbook of Attachment: Theory, Research, and Clinical Applications*. Edited by J. Cassidy and P. Shaver. New York: Guilford Press.

McCarty, M. E.; R. K. Clifton; and R. R. Collard. 1999. "Problem Solving in Infancy: The Emergence of an Action Plan," *Developmental Psychology*, Vol. 35, No. 4, 1091–1101.

Meisels, S. J., and others. 2003. *The Ounce Scale: Standards for the Developmental Profiles (Birth–42 Months)*. New York: Pearson Early Learning.

Melson, G., and A. Cohen. 1981. "Contextual Influences on Children's Activity: Sex Differences in Effects of Peer Presence and Interpersonal Attraction," *Genetic Psychology Monographs,* Vol. 103, 243–60.

Messinger, D., and A. Fogel. 2007. "The Interactive Development of Social Smiling," in *Advances in Child Development and Behavior* (Vol. 35). Edited by R. V. Kail. Burlington, MA: Elsevier.

Mesquita, B., and N. Frijda. 1992. "Cultural Variations in Emotions: A Review," *Psychological Bulletin,* Vol. 112, No. 2, 179–204.

Mueller, E., and T. Lucas. 1975. "A Developmental Analysis of Peer Interaction Among Toddlers," in *Friendship and Peer Relations.* Edited by M. Lewis and L. Rosenblum. New York: Wiley.

National Research Council and Institute of Medicine. 2000. *From Neurons to Neighborhoods: The Science of Early Childhood Development.* Committee on Integrating the Science of Early Childhood Development. Edited by J. P. Shonkoff and D. A. Phillips. Board on Children, Youth and Families, Commission on Behavioral and Social Sciences and Education. Washington, DC: National Academies Press.

National Scientific Council on the Developing Child. Winter, 2004. "Children's Emotional Development Is Built into the Architecture of Their Brains," *Working Paper* No. 2. http://www.developingchild.net (accessed on December 5, 2006)

Panksepp, J. 2001. The Long-Term Psychobiological Consequences of Infant Emotions: Prescriptions for the Twenty-First Century," *Infant Mental Health Journal,* Vol. 22, No. 1–2, 132–73.

Parks, S. 2004. *Inside HELP: Hawaii Early Learning Profile Administration and Reference Manual.* Palo Alto, CA: VORT Corporation.

Parritz, R. H. 1996. "A Descriptive Analysis of Toddler Coping in Challenging Circumstances," *Infant Behavior and Development,* Vol. 19, 171–80.

Pruett, K. D. 1999. *Me, Myself and I: How Children Build Their Sense of Self (18 to 36 Months).* New York: Goddard Press.

Quann, V., and C. Wien. 2006. "The Visible Empathy of Infants and Toddlers," *Young Children,* Vol. 61, No. 4, 22–29.

Raikes, H. 1996. "A Secure Base for Babies: Applying Attachment Concepts to the Infant Care Setting," *Young Children,* Vol. 51, No. 5, 59–67.

Raver, C. 2002. "Emotions Matter: Making the Case for the Role of Young Children's Emotional Development for Early School Readiness," *SRCD Social Policy Report,* Vol. 16, No. 3.

Ross, H. S., and B. D. Goldman. 1977. "Establishing New Social Relations in Infancy," in *Attachment Behavior.* Edited by T. Alloway, P. Pliner, and L. Krames. New York: Plenum Press.

Rothbart, M. K.; H. Ziaie; and C. G. O'Boyle. 1992. "Self-Regulation and Emotion in Infancy," in *Emotion and Its Regulation in Early Development* (No. 55). Edited by N. Eisenberg and R. Fabes. San Francisco: Jossey-Bass/Pfeiffer.

Ryalls, B.; R. Gul; and K. Ryalls. 2000. "Infant Imitation of Peer and Adult Models: Evidence for a Peer Model Advantage," *Merrill-Palmer Quarterly,* Vol. 46, No.1, 188–202.

Saarni, C., and others. 2006. "Emotional Development: Action, Communication, and Understanding," in *Handbook of Child Psychology* (Sixth edition), *Vol. 3, Social, Emotional, and Personality Development.* Edited by N. Eisenberg. Hoboken, NJ: John Wiley and Sons.

Schaffer, H. R., and P. E. Emerson. 1964. "The Development of Social Attachments in Infancy," *Monographs of the Society for Research in Child Development,* Vol. 29, No. 3.

Segal, M. 2004. "The Roots and Fruits of Pretending," in *Children's Play: The Roots of Reading.* Edited by E. F. Zigler, D. G. Singer, and S. J. Bishop-Josef. Washington, DC: Zero to Three Press.

Shonkoff, J. P. 2004. *Science, Policy and the Developing Child: Closing the Gap Between What We Know and What We Do.* Washington, DC: Ounce of Prevention Fund. http://www.ounceofprevention.org/downloads/publications/shonkoffweb.pdf (accessed on December 7, 2006)

Siegel, D. J. 1999. *The Developing Mind: How Relationships and the Brain Interact to Shape Who We Are.* New York: Guilford Press.

Squires, J.; D. Bricker; and E. Twombly. 2002. *The Ages & Stages Questionnaires: Social-Emotional. A Parent-Completed Child-Monitoring System for Social-Emotional Behaviors ASQ:SE.* User's Guide. Baltimore, MD: Paul H. Brookes Publishing.

Sroufe, L. A. 1979. "Socioemotional Development," in *Handbook of Infant Development.* Edited by J. Osofsky. New York: Wiley.

Stern, D. N. 1985. *The Interpersonal World of the Infant: A View from Psychoanalysis and Developmental Psychology.* New York: Basic Books.

Sternberg, C. R.; J. J. Campos; and R. N. Emde. 1983. "The Facial Expression of Anger in Seven-Month-Old Infants," *Child Development,* Vol. 54, 178–84.

Stipek, D. J.; J. H. Gralinski; and C. B. Kopp. 1990. "Self-Concept Development in the Toddler Years," *Developmental Psychology,* Vol. 26, No. 6, 972–77.

Taumoepeau, M., and T. Ruffman. 2008. "Stepping Stones to Others' Minds: Maternal Talk Relates to Child Mental State Language and Emotion Understanding at 15, 24, and 33 Months," *Child Development,* Vol. 79, No. 2, 284–302.

Teti, D. M. 1999. "Conceptualizations of Disorganization in the Preschool Years: An Integration," in *Attachment Disorganization.* Edited by J. Solomon and C. George. New York: Guilford Press.

Thelen, E., and A. Fogel. 1989. "Toward an Action-Based Theory of Infant Development," in *Action in Social Context: Perspectives on Early Development.* Edited by J. Lockman and N. Hazen. New York: Plenum Press.

Thompson, R. A. 1987. "Empathy and Emotional Understanding: The Early Development of Empathy," in *Empathy and Its Development.* Edited by N. Eisenberg and J. Strayer. New York: Cambridge University Press.

Thompson, R. A. 2006. "The Development of the Person: Social Understanding, Relationships, Self, Conscience," in *Handbook of Child Psychology* (Sixth edition), *Volume 3: Social, Emotional, and Personality Development.* Edited by N. Eisenberg. Hoboken, NJ: Wiley and Sons.

Thompson, R. A., and R. Goodvin. 2005. "The Individual Child: Temperament, Emotion, Self and Personality," in *Developmental Science: An Advanced Textbook* (Fifth edition). Edited by M. H. Bornstein and M. E. Lamb. Mahwah, NJ: Lawrence Erlbaum Associates.

Tronick, E. Z. 1989. "Emotions and Emotional Communication in Infants," *American Psychologist,* Vol. 44, No. 2, 112–19.

Tsai, J.; B. Knutson; and H. Fung. 2006. "Cultural Variation in Affect Valuation," *Journal of Personality and Social Psychology,* Vol. 90, No. 2, 288–307.

Tsai, J.; R. Levenson; and K. McCoy. 2006. "Cultural and Temperamental Variation in Emotional Response," *Emotion,* Vol. 6, No. 3, 484–97.

Tsai, J., and others. 2007. "Learning What Feelings to Desire: Socialization of Ideal Affect Through Children's Storybooks," *Personality and Social Psychology Bulletin,* Vol. 33, No. 1, 17–30.

Weinberg, M. K., and others. 1999. "Gender Differences in Emotional Expressivity and Self-Regulation During Early Infancy," *Developmental Psychology*, Vol. 35, No. 1, 175–88.

Wellman, H. M., and K. H. Lagattuta. 2000. "Developing Understandings of Mind," in *Understanding Other Minds: Perspectives from Developmental Cognitive Neuroscience*. Edited by S. Baron-Cohen, T. Tager-Flusberg, and D. J. Cohen. New York: Oxford University Press.

Wingert, P., and M. Brant. 2005. "Reading Your Baby's Mind," *Newsweek*, Aug. 15, 2005, 32–39.

Yuill, N. 1984. "Young Children's Coordination of Motive and Outcome in Judgments of Satisfaction and Morality," *British Journal of Developmental Psychology*, Vol. 2, 73–81.

Zahn-Waxler, C., and M. Radke-Yarrow. 1982. "The Development of Altruism: Alternative Research Strategies," in *The Development of Prosocial Behavior*. Edited by N. Eisenberg. New York: Academic Press.

Zahn-Waxler, C., and M. Radke-Yarrow. 1990. "The Origins of Empathetic Concern," *Motivation and Emotion*, Vol. 14, 107–30.

Zahn-Waxler, C., and others. 1992. "Development of Concern for Others," *Developmental Psychology*, Vol. 28, No. 1, 126–36.

Zahn-Waxler, C.; J. Robinson; and R. Emde. 1992. "Development of Empathy in Twins," *Developmental Psychology*, Vol. 28, No. 6, 1038–47.

Zero to Three. 2004. Infant and Early Childhood Mental Health: Promoting Healthy Social and Emotional Development. Fact Sheet, May 18, 2004. Washington, DC: Zero to Three. http://www.zerotothree.org/policy/ (accessed on December 7, 2006).

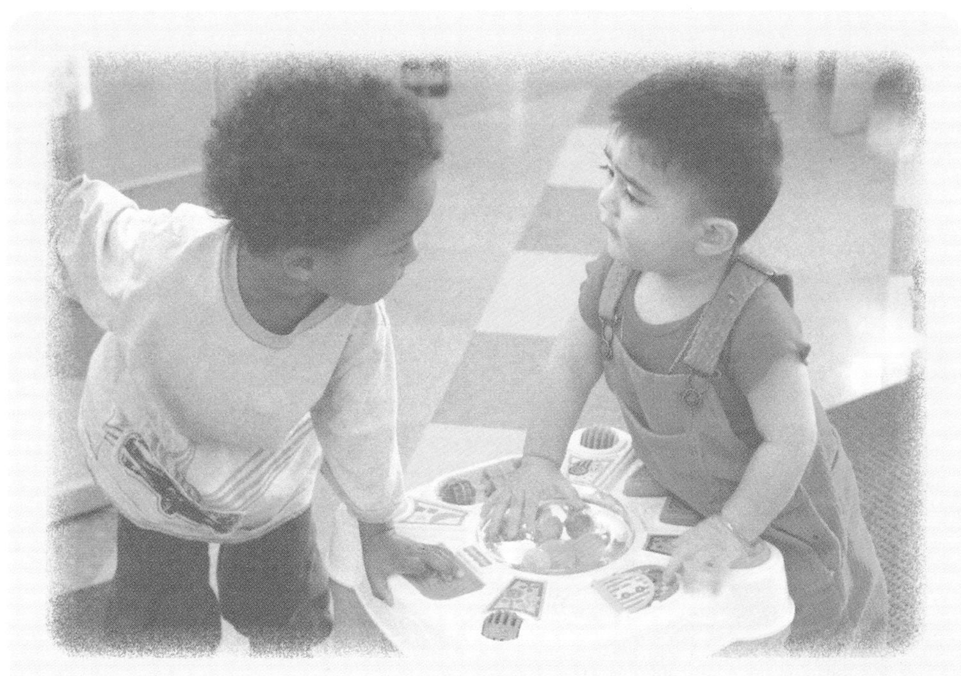

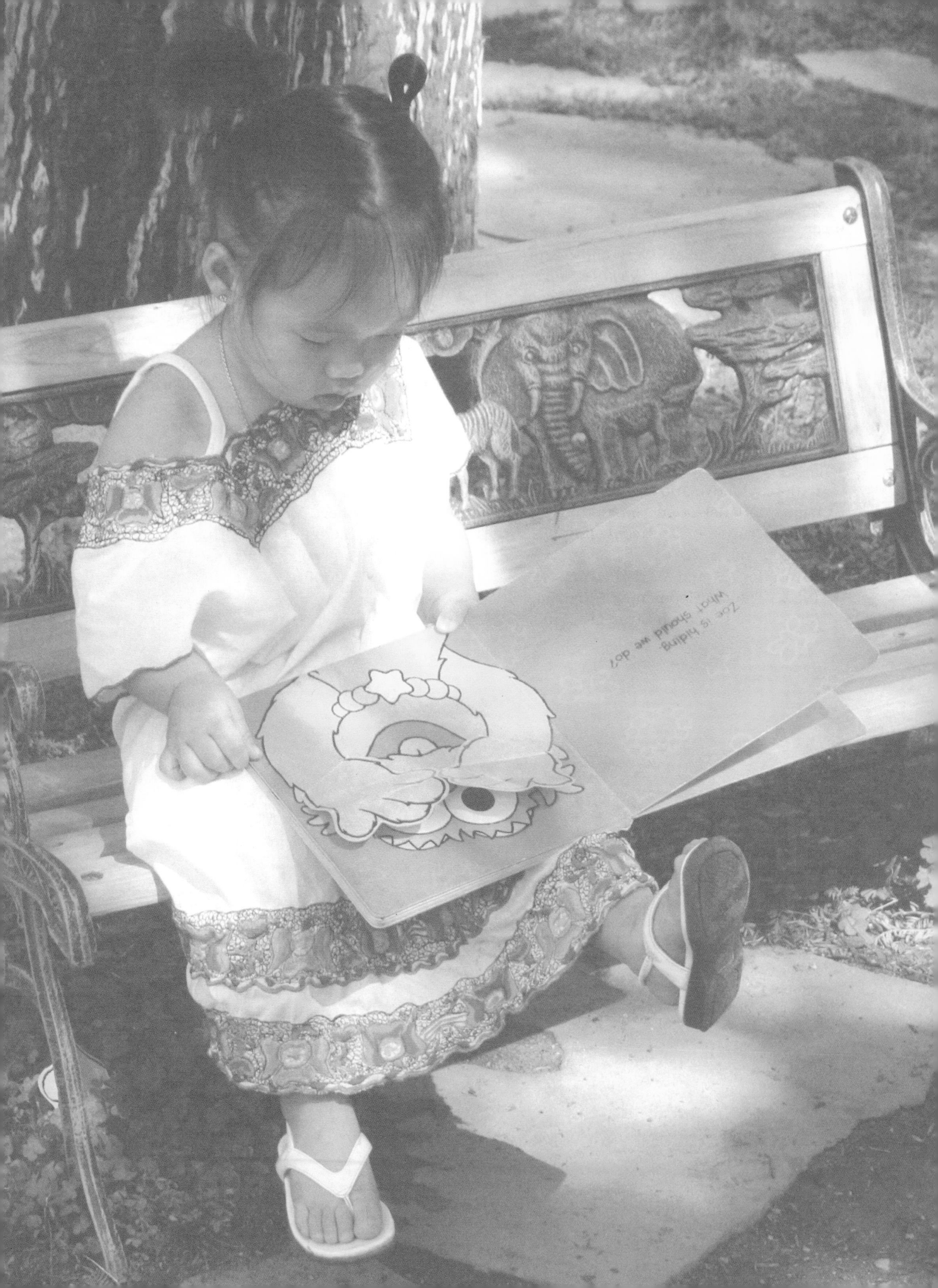
Zoe is hiding.
What should we do?

Language Development

"The acquisition of language and speech seems deceptively simple. Young children learn their mother tongue rapidly and effortlessly, from babbling at six months of age to full sentences by the end of three years, and follow the same developmental path regardless of culture." (Kuhl 2004, 831)

As is true of human development in infancy overall, language development occurs in the context of relationships. Emotion and language development in the early years are linked, as "much of the form and content of communication between infants and their caregivers in the first year of life depends upon affective expression" (Bloom and Capatides 1987, 1513). The relationship basis of early language development appears right at the beginning of life. Newborns prefer the sounds of their mothers' voices (DeCasper and Fifer 1980). They also prefer the language spoken by their mother during her pregnancy (Moon, Cooper, and Fifer 1993).

Adults typically modify their speech when communicating with young infants. Research suggests that infant-directed speech (also referred to as "parentese" or "motherese") has qualities, notably its pitch or tone and sing-song-like rhythm, that distinguish it from adult-directed speech (Cooper and others 1997). Preverbal infants communicate through eye contact, facial expressions, gestures, and sounds. Understanding language precedes speaking it (Bloom and others 1996). In addition, before being able to use language effectively, infants acquire some understanding of the social processes involved in communication. They learn about the social aspects of communication through engaging in turn-taking behavior in proto-conversations with their parents or infant care teachers. In proto-conversations, the adult usually says something to the preverbal infant, and the infant responds by making eye contact, cooing, smiling, showing lip and tongue movements, or waving arms. These "conversation-like" conversations go back and forth between the adult and the infant for several turns.

There is broad variability in language development in its pattern and pace (Bloom and Capatides 1987). However, the process of early language development is fundamentally the same across cultures and languages. In describing early language development, Kuhl (2002, 115) states: "One of the puzzles in language development is to explain the orderly transition that all infants go through during development. Infants the world over achieve certain milestones in linguistic development at roughly the same time, regardless of the language they are exposed to."

Perceptual processes play an important role in language development. As Gogate, Walker-Andrews, and Bahrick (2001, 13) note: "A diverse set of experimental findings suggests that early lexical comprehension owes much to infants' developing ability to perceive intersensory relations in auditory-visual events," [for example, speech]. Experience also affects language development from very early in life. One of the ways experience influences language development is through its impact on perception early in infancy. Prior to infants' first spoken words, or word comprehension, they have already "come to recognize the perceptual properties of their native language" (Kuhl 2002, 119). Infants are learning about the prosodic or sound characteristics of their native language: by nine months of age, English-speaking infants demonstrate a preference for the sound stress pattern characteristic of words in the English language (Jusczyk, Cutler, and Redanz 1993). Kuhl (2002, 112) concludes: "At age one—prior to the time infants begin to master higher levels of language, such as sound-meaning correspondences, contrastive phonology, and grammatical rules—infants' perceptual and perceptual-motor systems have been altered by linguistic experience. Phonetic perception has changed dramatically to conform to the native-language pattern, and language-specific speech production has emerged."

Receptive Language

Infants excel at detecting patterns in spoken language (Kuhl 2000). The literature indicates that infants' speech perception abilities are strong. Not only do infants understand more vocabulary than they are able to produce, but they also demonstrate awareness of the properties of the language or languages they are exposed to before they acquire words (Ingram 1999). During the first six months of life, infants are better than adults at perceiving various types of contrasts in speech (Plunkett and Schafer 1999). Infants improve in their ability to discriminate the sounds characteristic of their native language while losing their abilities to discriminate some sounds characteristic of languages other than their native language (Cheour and others 1998). According to Kuhl (2004), the way in which the infant's brain processes repeated experiences with speech explains language acquisition in a social and biological context. According to this view, from early infancy young children use a mental filter to orient, with greater efficiency and accuracy, to the speech sounds characteristic of their native language. This strategy enables infants to identify the phonemic units most useful to them in their native language and serves as a building block to later word acquisition (Kuhl 2004).

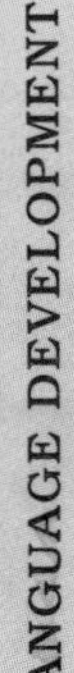

Expressive Language

Infants use their expressive language skills to make sounds or use gestures or speech to begin to communicate. Even preverbal infants use vocalizing or babbling to express themselves. They also imitate the sounds and rhythm of adult speech. As they develop, infants generate increasingly understandable sounds or verbal communication. They demonstrate their expressive language abilities by asking questions and responding to them and repeating of sounds or rhymes. Children typically acquire their first 50 words between the ages of one and two (Ingram 1999). Kuczaj (1999, 145) notes: "The 24-month-old child with a productive vocabulary between 50 and 600 words will easily quadruple or quintuple her vocabulary in the next year, and then add between 3000 and 4000 words per year to her productive vocabulary until she graduates from high school."

Infants' use of nonverbal gestures as a form of communication appears to be a typical feature of early language development, although there is considerable variability among children (Acredolo and Goodwyn 1988). The use of communicative gestures appears to generally precede the child's first words (Carpenter, Nagell, and Tomasello 1998). Commenting on the infant's motivation to use gestures, Acredolo and Goodwyn (1997, 30) state that the human infant has a special capacity to communicate with gestures. Acredolo and Goodwyn (1997) go on to say that typically developing infants seem so intent on communicating once they realize there is somebody out there "listening" that they find creative ways to do so before they have mastered words.

Communication Skills and Knowledge

Sensitivity to the timing of conversational exchanges has been demonstrated through research on back-and-forth communication involving young infants (Rochat, Querido, and Striano 1999). Infants use speech, gestures, and facial expressions as well as direct their attention to communicate to others. As they grow, they increasingly understand the rules or conventions of social communication. Infants also gain an expanded vocabulary that helps them express themselves through words. As they develop, infants benefit from communicating with both peers and adults, very different conversational partners. According to Pan and Snow (1999, 231), "Interaction with peers, who are less competent and usually less cooperative partners than adults, requires use of more sophisticated conversational skills, such as knowing how and when to interrupt, how to remedy overlaps and interruptions by others, and how to make topic-relevant moves." One type of environment that typically offers abundant opportunities for communication with both adult and child conversational partners is high-quality child care settings.

Interest in Print

Infants show an interest in print at first through physically exploring, such as putting books in their mouths, handling books, or focusing on print in the environment around them. Turning the pages of books, looking at books or pictures, asking for a favorite book or telling a favorite story with an adult are other indicators of interest in print. As infants grow older, making intentional marks on paper with a crayon or marker, pretending to read and write, repeating stories, repeating rhymes, recognizing images in books, noticing common symbols and words, and enjoying books are all related to interest in print. Interest in print can be considered one aspect of emergent literacy, the idea that literacy develops from early childhood rather than something that becomes relevant only upon school entry (Whitehurst and Lonigan 1998). Because early experiences with print contribute to later literacy, shared book reading is recommended as a valuable way to promote emergent literacy (Whitehurst and Lonigan 1998).

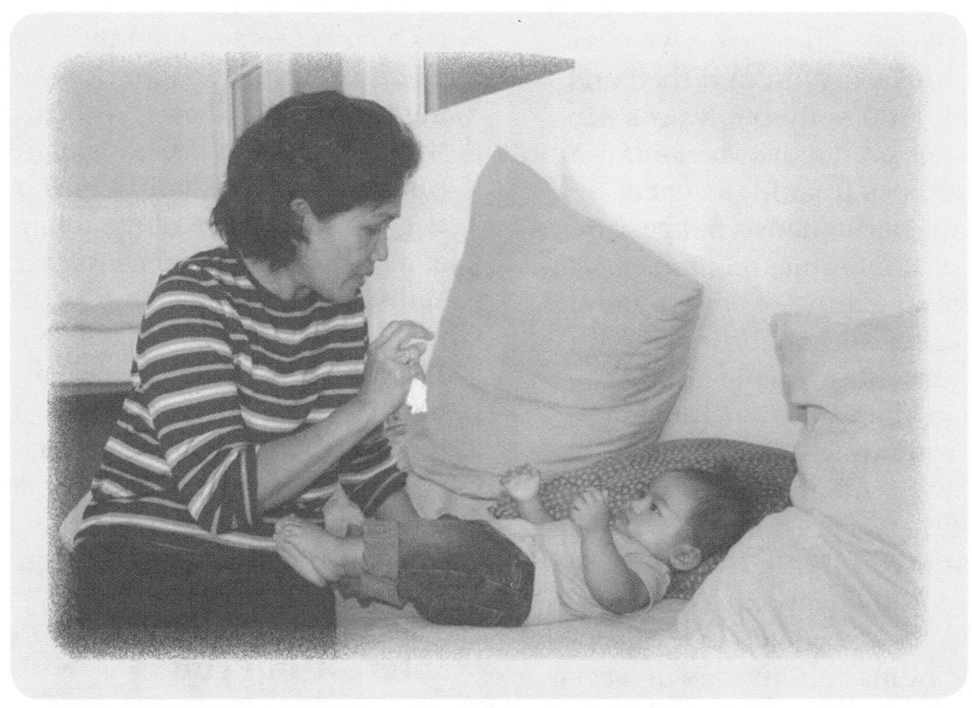

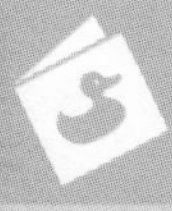

Foundation: Receptive Language

The developing ability to understand words and increasingly complex utterances

8 months	*18 months*	*36 months*
At around eight months of age, children show understanding of a small number of familiar words and react to the infant care teacher's overall tone of voice.	At around 18 months of age, children show understanding of one-step requests that have to do with the current situation.	At around 36 months of age, children demonstrate understanding of the meaning of others' comments, questions, requests, or stories. (By 36 mos.; American Academy of Pediatrics 2004, 307)
For example, the child may:	**For example, the child may:**	**For example, the child may:**
• Smile and look toward the door when the infant care teacher says, "Daddy's here." (Scaled score of 10 for 7:16–8:15 mos.; Bayley 2006, 87) • Wave arms and kick legs in excitement when the infant care teacher says, "bottle." (8 mos.; Meisels and others 2003, 18) • Smile when the infant care teacher uses baby talk and make a worried face when she uses a stern voice. (8 mos.; Meisels and others 2003, 18; by end of 7 mos.; American Academy of Pediatrics 2004)	• Go to the cubby when the infant care teacher says that it is time to put on coats to go outside. (Scaled score of 10 for 17:16 to 18:15 mos.; Bayley 2006, 90; 12–18 mos.; Lerner and Ciervo 2003; 12 mos.; Coplan 1993, 2; by 24 mos.; American Academy of Pediatrics 2004; 12 mos.; Coplan 1993, 2; 24 mos.; Meisels and others 2003, 46) • Cover up the doll when the infant care teacher says, "Cover the baby with the blanket." (Scaled score of 10 for 17:16–18:15 mos.; Bayley 2006, 90; 12–18 mos.; Lerner and Ciervo 2003; 12 mos.; Coplan 1993, 2; by 24 mos.; American Academy of Pediatrics 2004) • Go to the sink when the infant care teacher says that it is time to wash hands. (Scaled score of 10 for 17:16–18:15 mos.; Bayley 2006, 90; 12–18 mos.; Lerner and Ciervo 2003; 12 mos.; Coplan 1993, 2; by 24 mos.; American Academy of Pediatrics 2004; 24 mos.; Meisels and others 2003, 46) • Get a tissue when the infant care teacher says, "Please go get a tissue. We need to wipe your nose." (18 mos.; Meisels and others 2003, 36)	• Look for a stuffed bear when the infant care teacher asks, "Where's your bear?" (24–36 mos.; Coplan 1993, 2–3; scaled score of 10 for 34:16–35:15; Bayley 2006) • Get the bin of blocks when the infant care teacher asks what the child wants to play with. (24–36 mos.; Coplan 1993, 2–3; scaled score of 10 for 34:16–35:15; Bayley 2006) • Show understanding of words such as *no, not,* and *don't,* and utterances such as when the infant care teacher says, "There's no more milk," or "Those don't go there." (24–36 mos.; Parks 2004, p. 99) • Know the names of most objects in the immediate environment. (By 36 mos.; American Academy of Pediatrics 2004) • Understand requests that include simple prepositions, such as, "Please put your cup on the table," or "Please get your blanket out of your back-pack." (By 36 mos.; Coplan 1993, 2; by 36 mos.; American Academy of Pediatrics 2004; 24–27 mos.; Parks 2004, 97) • Laugh when an adult tells a silly joke or makes up rhymes with nonsense "words." (By 36 mos.; American Academy of Pediatrics 2004, 307) • Show understanding of the meaning of a story by laughing at the funny parts or by asking questions. (By 36 mos.; American Academy of Pediatrics 2004, 307)

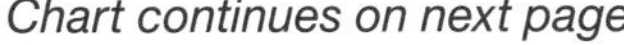
Chart continues on next page.

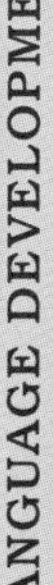

Receptive Language

Behaviors leading up to the foundation (4 to 7 months)	Behaviors leading up to the foundation (9 to 17 months)	Behaviors leading up to the foundation (19 to 35 months)
During this period, the child may: • Vocalize in response to the infant care teacher's speech. (3–6 mos.; Parks 2004) • Quiet down when hearing the infant care teacher's voice. (3–6 mos.; Parks 2004) • Turn toward the window when hearing a fire truck drive by. (4–6 mos.; Coplan 1993, 2) • Quiet down and focus on the infant care teacher as he talks to the child during a diaper change. (4 mos.; Meisels and others 2003, 10) • Look at or turn toward the infant care teacher who says the child's name. (Mean for 5 mos.; Bayley 2006, 86; by 7 mos.; American Academy of Pediatrics 2004, 209; 9 mos.; Coplan 1993, 2; 12 mos.; Meisels and others 2003, 27; 5–7 mos.; Parks 2004)	During this period, the child may: • Follow one-step simple requests if the infant care teacher also uses a gesture to match the verbal request, such as pointing to the blanket when asking the child to get it. (9 mos.; Coplan 1993, 2) • Look up and momentarily stop reaching into the mother's purse when she says "no no." (9–12 mos.; Parks 2004, 95) • Show understanding of the names for most familiar objects and people. (Scaled score of 10 for 16:16–17:15 mos.; Bayley 2006, 90; 8–12 mos.; Parks 2004, 94)	During this period, the child may: • Show understanding of pronouns, such as *he, she, you, me, I,* and *it;* for example, by touching own nose when the infant care teacher says, "Where's your nose?" and then touching the infant care teacher's nose when he says, "And where's my nose?" (19 mos.; Hart and Risley 1999, 61; 20–24 mos.; Parks 2004, 96) • Follow two-step requests about unrelated events, such as, "Put the blocks away and then go pick out a book." (24 mos.; Coplan 1993, 2; by 24 mos.; American Academy of Pediatrics 2004, 270; 24–29 mos.; Parks 2004, 104; three-part command by 36 mos.; American Academy of Pediatrics 2004, 307) • Answer adults' questions; for example, communicate "apple" when a parent asks what the child had for snack. (28 mos.; Hart and Risley 1999, 95)

Foundation: Expressive Language

The developing ability to produce the sounds of language and use vocabulary and increasingly complex utterances

8 months	*18 months*	*36 months*
At around eight months of age, children experiment with sounds, practice making sounds, and use sounds or gestures to communicate needs, wants, or interests.	At around 18 months of age, children say a few words and use conventional gestures to tell others about their needs, wants, and interests. (By 15 to 18 mos.; American Academy of Pediatrics 2004 270; Coplan 1993, 1; Hulit and Howard 2006, 142)	At around 36 months of age, children communicate in a way that is understandable to most adults who speak the same language they do. Children combine words into simple sentences and demonstrate the ability to follow some grammatical rules of the home language. (By 36 mos.; American Academy of Pediatrics 2004, 307; 30–36 mos.; Parks 2004; 24–36 mos.; Lerner and Ciervo 2003; by 36 mos.; Hart and Risley 1999, 67)
For example, the child may:	**For example, the child may:**	**For example, the child may:**
• Vocalize to get the infant care teacher's attention. (6.5–8 mos.; Parks 2004) • Repeat sounds when babbling, such as "da da da da" or "ba ba ba ba." (By 7 mos.; American Academy of Pediatrics 2004, 209; 6–7 mos.; Hulit and Howard 2006, 122; scaled score of 10 for 7:16–8:15 on Bayley 2006, 106; 4–6.5 mos.; Parks 2004; 6 mos.; Locke 1993) • Wave to the infant care teacher when he waves and says, "bye-bye" as he leaves for his break. (6–9 mos.; Parks 2004, 121) • Lift arms to the infant care teacher to communicate a desire to be held. (7–9 mos.; Coplan 1993, 3; 5–9 mos.; Parks 2004, 121)	• Look at a plate of crackers, then at the infant care teacher, and communicate "more." (Scaled score of 10 for 16:16–17:15; Bayley 2006; 14–20 mos.; Parks 2004) • Point to an airplane in the sky and look at the infant care teacher. (17.5–18.5 mos.; Parks 2004, 123) • Use the same word to refer to similar things, such as "milk" while indicating the pitcher, even though it is filled with juice. (18 mos.; Meisels and others 2003, p. 37) • Use two words together, such as "Daddy give." (18 mos.; National Research Council and Institute of Medicine 2000, 127) • Shake head "no" when offered more food. (18 mos.; Meisels and others 2003, 37) • Jabber a string of sounds into the toy telephone. (18 mos.; Meisels and others 2003, 37) • Gesture "all gone" by twisting wrists to turn hands up and down when finished eating lunch. (12–19 mos.; Parks 2004, 122) • Use made-up "words" to refer to objects or experiences that only familiar adults will know the meaning of; for example "wo-wo" when wanting to go next door to visit the puppy. (12–22 mos.; Hulit and Howard 2006, p. 130)	• Use the past tense, though not always correctly; for example, "Daddy goed to work," "She falled down." (27–30 mos.; Hulit and Howard 2006, 182; 30–36 mos.; Parks 2004; 28 mos.; Hart and Risley 1999, 95 and 129–30) • Use the possessive, though not always correctly; for example, "That's you car" or "Her Megan." (Scaled score of 10 for 34:16–35:15; Bayley 2006) • Use a few prepositions, such as "on" the table. (33-35.5 mos.; Parks 2004, p. 116) • Talk about what she will do in the future, such as "I gonna get a kitty." (33–36 mos.; Hart and Risley 1999, 131) • Use 300–1000 words. (35+ mos.; Parks 2004, 116) • Use the plural form of nouns, though not always correctly; for example, "mans," and "mouses." (By 36 mos.; American Academy of Pediatrics 2004, 307; 28 mos.; Hart and Risley 1999, 95) • Express, "Uncle is coming to pick me up." (36 mos.; Hoff 2005)

Chart continues on next page.

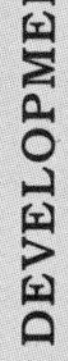

Expressive Language

Behaviors leading up to the foundation (4 to 7 months)	Behaviors leading up to the foundation (9 to 17 months)	Behaviors leading up to the foundation (19 to 35 months)
During this period, the child may: • Squeal when excited. (5 mos.; Lerner and Ciervo 2003; by 7 mos.; American Academy of Pediatrics 2004, 209) • Make an angry noise when another child takes a toy. (5–6 mos.; Parks 2004) • Make a face of disgust to tell the infant care teacher that she does not want any more food. (6–9 mos.; Lerner and Ciervo 2003)	During this period, the child may: • Babble using the sounds of his home language. (6–10 mos.; Cheour and others 1998) • Consistently use utterances to refer to favorite objects or experiences that only familiar adults know the meaning of; for example, "ba ba ba ba" for blanket. (9 mos.; Bates, Camaioni, and Volterra 1975; 12 mos.; Coplan 1993, 3; 12 mos.; Davies 2004, 166; 9–10 mos.; Hulit and Howard 2006, 123) • Express "Mama" or "Dada" when the mother or father, respectively, enters the room. (10 mos.; Coplan 1993, 1) • Say a first word clearly enough that the infant care teacher can understand the word within the context; for example, "gih" for give, "see," "dis" for this, "cookie," "doggie," "uh oh" and "no." (Mean age 11 mos.; Hart and Risley 1999, 56) • Name a few familiar favorite objects. (Around 12 mos.; Coplan 1993, 3; mean age 13 mos., range 9–16 mos.; Hulit and Howard 2006, 132; between 10 and 15 mos.; National Research Council and Institute of Medicine 2000, 127) • Change tone when babbling, so that the child's babbles sound more and more like adult speech. (By 12 mos.; American Academy of Pediatrics 2004; 7.5–12 mos.; Parks, 2004; 7–8 mos.; Hulit and Howard 2006, 123) • Use expressions; for example, "uh oh" when milk spills or when something falls off the table. (12.5–14.5 mos.; Parks 2004) • Say "up" and lift arms to be picked up by the infant care teacher. (Scaled score of 9 for 16:16–17:15 mos.; Bayley 2006, 108; 12–14 mos.; Parks 2004, 132)	During this period, the child may: • Tend to communicate about objects, actions, and events that are in the here and now. (12–22 mos.; Hulit and Howard 2006, 141) • Use some words to refer to more than one thing; for example, "night-night" to refer to bedtime or to describe darkness. (12–22 mos.; Hulit and Howard 2006, 132) • Use many new words each day. (18–20 mos.; Coplan, 1993, 1; 18–24 mos.; Hulit and Howard 2006, 137) • Begin to combine a few words into mini-sentences to express wants, needs, or interests; for example, "more milk," "big doggie," "no night-night" or "go bye-bye." (18–20 mos.; Coplan 1993, 1; 24 mos.; Meisels and others 2003, 47; by 24 mos.; American Academy of Pediatrics 2004, 270; 18–24 mos.; Hulit and Howard 2006, 143; scaled score of 10 for 32:16–33:15; Bayley 2006, 114; 20.5–24 mos.; Parks 2004, 133) • Have a vocabulary of about 80 words. (19 mos.; Hart and Risley 1999, 61) • Start adding articles before nouns, such as, "a book" or "the cup." (20 mos.; Hart and Risley 1999, 63) • Use own name when referring to self. (18-24 mos.; Parks 2004) • Ask questions with raised intonations at the end, such as "Doggy go?" (22–26 mos.; Hulit and Howard 2006, 144) • Communicate using sentences of three to five words, such as "Daddy go store?" or "Want more rice." (30 mos.; Coplan 1993, 1; 25 mos.; Hart and Risley 1999, 63)

Foundation: Communication Skills and Knowledge

The developing ability to communicate nonverbally and verbally

8 months	18 months	36 months
At around eight months of age, children participate in back-and-forth communication and games.	At around 18 months of age, children use conventional gestures and words to communicate meaning in short back-and-forth interactions and use the basic rules of conversational turn-taking when communicating. (Bloom, Rocissano, and Hood 1976)	At around 36 months of age, children engage in back-and-forth conversations that contain a number of turns, with each turn building upon what was said in the previous turn. (Hart and Risley 1999, 122)
For example, the child may:	**For example, the child may:**	**For example, the child may:**
• Put arms up above head when the infant care teacher says, "soooo big." (8 mos.; Meisels and others 2003, 19) • Try to get the infant care teacher to play peek-a-boo by hiding her face behind a blanket, uncovering her face, and laughing. (8 mos.; Meisels and others 2003, 19) • Pull the infant care teacher's hands away from his face during a game of peek-a-boo. (Scaled score of 11 for 7:16–8:15 mos.; Bayley 2006, 106) • Try to clap hands to get the infant care teacher to continue playing pat-a-cake. (8 mos.; Meisels and others 2003, 19) • Make sounds when the infant care teacher is singing a song. (8 mos.; Meisels and others 2003, 19) • Interact with the infant care teacher while singing a song with actions or while doing finger plays. (Scaled score of 11 for 8:16–9:15 mos.; Bayley 2006)	• Respond to the infant care teacher's initiation of conversation through vocalizations or nonverbal communication. (12–19 mos.; Hart and Risley 1999, 37) • Initiate interactions with the infant care teacher by touching, vocalizing, or offering a toy. (12–19 mos.; Hart and Risley 1999, 37) • Jabber into a toy phone and then pause, as if to listen to someone on the other end. (18 mos.; Meisels and others 2003, 37) • Shake head or express "no" when the infant care teacher asks if the child is ready to go back inside. (18 mos.; Meisels and others 2003, 37) • Respond to the infant care teacher's comment about a toy with an additional, but related, action or comment about the same toy; for example, make a barking sound when the infant care teacher pats a toy dog and says, "Nice doggie." (By 18 mos.; Bloom, Rocissano, and Hood 1976)	• Persist in trying to get the infant care teacher to respond by repeating, speaking more loudly, expanding on what the child said, or touching the infant care teacher. (After 30 mos.; Hart and Risley 1999, 38) • Repeat part of what the adult just said in order to continue the conversation. (31–34 mos.; Hulit and Howard 2006, 186; by 24 mos.; American Academy of Pediatrics 2004) • Make comments in a conversation that the other person has difficulty understanding; for example, suddenly switch topics or use pronouns without making clear what is being talked about. (31–34 mos.; Hulit and Howard 2006, 192) • Answer adults' questions, such as "What's that?" and "Where did it go?" (31–34 mos.; Hulit and Howard 2006, 185; 24–36 mos.; Parks 2004) • Begin to create understandable topics for a conversation partner. • Sometimes get frustrated if the infant care teacher does not understand what the child is trying to communicate. (28.5–36 mos.; Parks 2004, 129) • Participate in back-and-forth interaction with the infant care teacher by speaking, giving feedback, and adding to what was originally said. (29–36 mos.; Hart and Risley 1999, 36, 39–40)

Chart continues on next page.

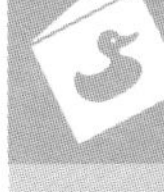

Communication Skills and Knowledge

Behaviors leading up to the foundation (4 to 7 months)	Behaviors leading up to the foundation (9 to 17 months)	Behaviors leading up to the foundation (19 to 35 months)
During this period, the child may: • Respond with babbling when the infant care teacher asks a question. (Hart and Risley 1999, 55) • Laugh when a parent nuzzles her face in the child's belly, vocalizes expectantly when she pulls back, and laugh when she nuzzles again. (3–6 mos.; Parks 2004, 11) • Move body in a rocking motion to get the infant care teacher to continue rocking. (4-5 mos.; Parks 2004, 57) • Babble back and forth with the infant care teacher during diaper change. (5.5–6.5 mos.; Parks 2004, 125)	During this period, the child may: • Copy the infant care teacher in waving "bye-bye" to a parent as he leaves the room. (Scaled score of 9 for 12:16–13:15 mos.; Bayley 2006, No. 14, 88; 8 mos.; Meisels and others 2003, 19) • Purse lips after hearing and seeing the infant care teacher make a sputtering sound with her lips. (9 mos.; Apfel and Provence 2001) • Repeat the last word in an adult's question in order to continue the conversation; for example, saying "dat" after the infant care teacher asks, "What is that?" (11–16 mos.; Hart and Risley 1999, 83) • Respond with "yes" or "no" when asked a simple question. (11–16 mos.; Hart and Risley 1999, 83) • Hold out a toy for the infant care teacher to take and then reach out to accept it when the infant care teacher offers it back. (12–15 mos.; Parks 2004, 122) • Show an understanding that a conversation must build on what the other partner says; for example, expressing, "bear" when the infant care teacher points to the stuffed bear and asks, "What's that?" (16 mos.; Hart and Risley 1999, 81) • Initiate back-and-forth interaction with the infant care teacher by babbling and then waiting for the infant care teacher to respond before babbling again. (11–19 mos.; Hart and Risley 1999, 77; 12 mos.; Meisels and others 2003, 27) • Say "mmm" when eating, after a parent says, "mmm." (11–19 mos.; Hart and Risley 1999, 78)	During this period, the child may: • Ask and answer simple questions, such as "What's that?" (19 mos.; Hart and Risley 1999, 61) • Say, "huh?" when interacting with the infant care teacher to keep interaction going. (19 mos.; Hart and Risley 1999, 62) • Repeat or add on to what she just said if the infant care teacher does not respond right away. (20–28 mos.; Hart and Risley 1999, 105) • Engage in short back-and-forth interactions with a family member by responding to comments, questions, and prompts. (20–28 mos.; Hart and Risley 1999, 39) • Respond almost immediately after a parent finishes talking in order to continue the interaction. (20–28 mos.; Hart and Risley 1999, 97) • Get frustrated if the infant care teacher does not understand what the child is trying to communicate. (24–28.5 mos.; Parks 2004) • Attempt to continue conversation, even when the adult does not understand him right away, by trying to use different words to communicate the meaning. (27–30 mos.; Hulit and Howard 2006, 182) • Sustain conversation about one topic for one or two turns, usually about something that is in the here and now. (20–28 mos.; Hart and Risley 1999, 107; 27–30 mos.; Hulit and Howard 2006, 182) • Respond verbally to adults' questions or comments. (27–30 mos.; Hulit and Howard 2006, 182)

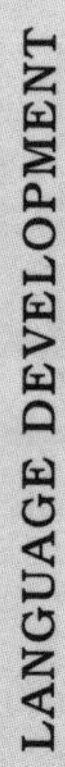

Foundation: Interest in Print

The developing interest in engaging with print in books and in the environment

8 months	18 months	36 months
At around eight months of age, children explore books and show interest in adult-initiated literacy activities, such as looking at photos and exploring books together with an adult. (Scaled score of 10 for 7:16–8:15 mos.; Bayley 2006, 57; infants; National Research Council 1999, 28)	At around 18 months of age, children listen to the adult and participate while being read to by pointing, turning pages, or making one- or two-word comments. Children actively notice print in the environment.	At around 36 months of age, children show appreciation for books and initiate literacy activities: listening, asking questions, or making comments while being read to; looking at books on their own; or making scribble marks on paper and pretending to read what is written. (Schickedanz and Casbergue 2004, 11)
For example, the child may:	**For example, the child may:**	**For example, the child may:**
• Point to or indicate an object that he would like the infant care teacher to pay attention to. • Look intently at photographs of classmates when the infant care teacher talks about the pictures. (8–9 mos.; Parks 2004, 71) • Look at pictures that a parent points to while reading a storybook. (Scaled score of 10 for 7:16–8:15 mos.; Bayley 2006, 57; infants; National Research Council 1999, 28) • Hold a book and try to turn the pages. (Scaled score of 10 for 7:16–8:15 mos.; Bayley 2006, 57)	• Attempt to turn the pages of a paper book, sometimes turning more than one page at a time. (15–18 mos.; Parks 2004) • Pretend to read the back of a cereal box while sitting at the kitchen table in the house area. (15–18 mos.; Parks 2004, 27) • Recognize a favorite book by its cover. (Toddler; National Research Council 1999, 28) • Pull the infant care teacher by the hand to the bookshelf, point, and express "book" to get the infant care teacher to read a story. (12–18 mos.; Lerner and Ciervo 2003) • Point to or indicate a familiar sign in the neighborhood.	• Enjoy both being read to and looking at books by himself. (30–36 mos.; Parks 2004) • Pretend to read books to stuffed animals by telling a story that is related to the pictures and turning the book around to show the picture to the stuffed animals, just as the infant care teacher does when reading to a small group of children. (Ehri and Sweet 1991, 199; 24–36 mos.; Sulzby 1985) • Talk about the trip to the library and ask about the next trip. (35 mos.; Hart and Risley 1999, 128) • Recite much of a favorite book from memory while "reading" it to others or self. (36 mos.; National Research Council 1999, 28) • Try to be careful with books. (By 36 mos.; National Research Council 1999, 3)

Chart continues on next page.

Interest in Print

Behaviors leading up to the foundation (4 to 7 months)	Behaviors leading up to the foundation (9 to 17 months)	Behaviors leading up to the foundation (19 to 35 months)
During this period, the child may: • Chew on a board book. (International Reading Association and the National Association for the Education of Young Children 1998, 198; 3–6 mos.; Parks 2004)	During this period, the child may: • Try to turn the pages of a paper book, turning several pages at one time. (scaled score of 10 for 9:16–10:15 mos.; Bayley 2006, 128) • Scribble with a crayon. (Scaled score of 10 for 12:16–13:15 mos.; Bayley 2006, 129) • Smile and point to or indicate pictures of favorite animals in a book. (10–14 mos.; Parks 2004) • Help the infant care teacher turn a page of a book. (14–15 mos.; Parks 2004) • Use an open hand to pat a picture while reading with a family member. (14–15 mos.; Parks 2004)	During this period, the child may: • Move behind the infant care teacher in order to look over her shoulder at the pictures, when there are several children crowded around. (18–24 mos.; Parks 2004, 68) • Turn the pages of a book one by one. (18–24 mos.; Parks 2004) • Listen as a family member reads short picture books aloud. (Scaled score of 10 for 21:15–22:16 mos.; Bayley 2006, 67; 27–30 mos.; Parks 2004) • Ask a question about a story; for example, "Bear go?" while turning from one page to the next. (24 mos.; Meisels and others 2003, 47)

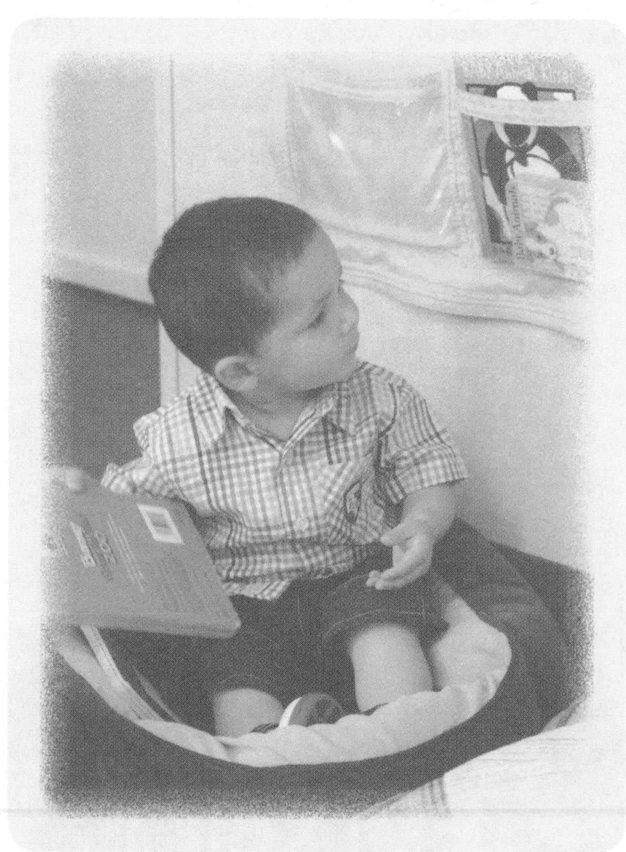

References

Acredolo, L., and S. Goodwyn. 1988. "Symbolic Gesturing in Normal Infants," *Child Development,* Vol. 59, 450–66.

Acredolo, L., and S. Goodwyn. 1997. "Furthering our Understanding of What Humans Understand," *Human Development,* Vol. 40, 25–31.

American Academy of Pediatrics. 2004. *Caring for Your Baby and Young Child: Birth to Age 5* (Fourth edition). Edited by S. P. Shelov and R. E. Hannemann. New York: Bantam Books.

Apfel, N. H., and S. Provence. 2001. *Manual for the Infant-Toddler and Family Instrument (ITFI).* Baltimore, MD: Paul H. Brookes Publishing.

Bates, E.; L. Camaioni; and V. Volterra. 1975. " The Acquisition of Performatives Prior to Speech," *Merrill-Palmer Quarterly,* Vol. 21, 205–26.

Bayley, N. 2006. *Bayley Scales of Infant and Toddler Development* (Third edition). San Antonio, TX: Harcourt Assessment Inc.

Bloom, L., and J. Capatides. 1987. "Expression of Affect and the Emergence of Language," *Child Development,* Vol. 58, 1513–22.

Bloom, L., and others. 1996. "Early Conversations and Word Learning: Contributions from Child and Adult," *Child Development,* Vol. 67, 3154–75.

Bloom, L.; L. Rocissano; and L. Hood. 1976. "Adult-Child Discourse: Developmental Interaction Between Information Processing and Linguistic Knowledge," *Cognitive Psychology,* Vol. 8, 521–52.

Carpenter, M.; K. Nagell; and M. Tomasello. 1998. "Social Cognition, Joint Attention, and Communicative Competence from 9 to 15 Months of Age," *Monographs of the Society for Research in Child Development,* Vol. 63, Serial No. 255, No. 4, 1–33.

Cheour, M., and others. 1998. "Development of Language-Specific Phoneme Representations in the Infant Brain," *Nature Neuroscience,* Vol. 1, 351–53.

Cooper, R. P., and others. 1997. "The Development of Infants' Preference for Motherese," *Infant Behavior and Development,* Vol. 20, No. 4, 477–88.

Coplan, J. 1993. *Early Language Milestone Scale: Examiner's Manual* (Second edition). Austin, TX: Pro-ed.

Davies, D. 2004. *Child Development: A Practitioner's Guide* (Second edition). New York: Guilford Press.

DeCasper, A., and W. Fifer. 1980. "On Human Bonding: Newborns Prefer Their Mothers' Voices," *Science,* Vol. 208, 1174–76.

Ehri, L., and J. Sweet. 1991. "Fingerpoint-Reading of Memorized Text: What Enables Beginners to Process the Print?" *Reading Research Quarterly,* Vol. 26, 442–62.

Gogate, L.; A. Walker-Andrews; and L. Bahrick. 2001. "The Intersensory Origins of Word Comprehension: An Ecological-Dynamic Systems View," *Developmental Science,* Vol. 4, No. 1, 1–37.

Hart, B., and T. R. Risley. 1999. *The Social World of Children: Learning to Talk.* Baltimore, MD: Paul H. Brookes Publishing Co.

Hoff, E. 2005. *Language Development* (Third edition). Belmont, CA: Wadsworth/Thomson Learning.

Hulit, L. M., and M. R. Howard. 2006. *Born to Talk: An Introduction to Speech and Language Development.* New York: Pearson Education, Inc.

Ingram, D. 1999. "Phonological Acquisition" in *The Development of Language.* Edited by M. Barrett. East Sussex, UK: Psychology Press.

International Reading Association and the National Association for the Education of Young Children. 1998. "Learning to Read and Write: Developmentally Appropriate Practices for Young Children," *The Reading Teacher,* Vol. 52, No. 2, 193–216.

Jusczyk, J.; A. Cutler; and N. J. Redanz. 1993. "Infants' Preference for the Predominant Stress Patterns of English Words," *Child Development,* Vol. 64, 675–87.

Kuczaj, S. 1999. "The World of Words: Thoughts on the Development of a Lexicon," in *The Development of Language.* Edited by M. Barrett. East Sussex, UK: Psychology Press.

Kuhl, P. K. 2000. "A New View of Language Acquisition," *Proceedings of the National Academy of Sciences of the United States,* Vol. 97, No. 22, 11850–857.

Kuhl, P. K. 2002. "Speech, Language and Developmental Change," in *Emerging Cognitive Abilities in Early Infancy.* Edited by F. Lacerda, C. von Hofsten, and M. Heimann. Mahwah, NJ: Lawrence Erlbaum Associates.

Kuhl, P. K. 2004. "Early Language Acquisition: Cracking the Speech Code," *Nature Reviews Neuroscience,* Vol. 5, 831–43.

Lerner, C., and L. A. Ciervo. 2003. *Healthy Minds: Nurturing Children's Development from 0 to 36 Months.* Washington, DC: Zero to Three Press and American Academy of Pediatrics.

Locke, J. L. 1993. *The Child's Path to Spoken Language.* Cambridge, MA: Harvard University Press.

Meisels, S. J., and others. 2003. *The Ounce Scale: Standards for the Developmental Profiles (Birth–42 Months).* New York: Pearson Early Learning.

Moon, C.; R. Cooper; and W. Fifer. 1993. "Two-Day-Olds Prefer their Native Language," *Infant Behavior and Development,* Vol. 16, 495–500.

National Research Council. 1999. *Starting Out Right: A Guide to Promoting Children's Reading Success.* Washington, DC: National Academy Press.

National Research Council and Institute of Medicine. 2000. *From Neurons to Neighborhoods: The Science of Early Childhood Development.* Committee on Integrating the Science of Early Childhood Development. Edited by J. P. Shonkoff and D. A. Phillips. Washington, DC: National Academies Press.

Pan, B., and C. Snow. 1999. "The Development of Conversational and Discourse Skills," in *The Development of Language.* Edited by M. Barrett. East Sussex, UK: Psychology Press.

Parks, S. 2004. *Inside HELP: Hawaii Early Learning Profile: Administration and Reference Manual.* Palo Alto, CA: VORT Corporation.

Plunkett, K., and G. Schafer. 1999. "Early Speech Perception and Word Learning," in *The Development of Language.* Edited by M. Barrett. East Sussex, UK: Psychology Press.

Rochat, P.; J. Querido; and T. Striano. 1999. "Emerging Sensitivity to the Timing and Structure of Protoconversation in Early Infancy," *Developmental Psychology,* Vol. 35, No. 4, 950–57.

Schickedanz, J. A., and R. M. Casbergue. 2004. *Writing in Preschool: Learning to Orchestrate Meaning and Marks.* Newark, DE: International Reading Association.

Sulzby, E. 1985. "Children's Emergent Reading of Favorite Storybooks: A Developmental Study," *Reading Research Quarterly,* Vol. 20, 458–81.

Whitehurst, G., and C. Lonigan. 1998. "Child Development and Emergent Literacy," *Child Development,* Vol. 69, No. 3, 848–72.

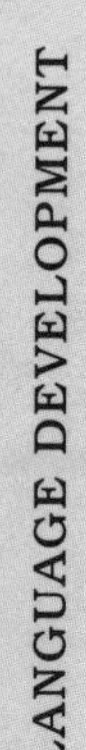

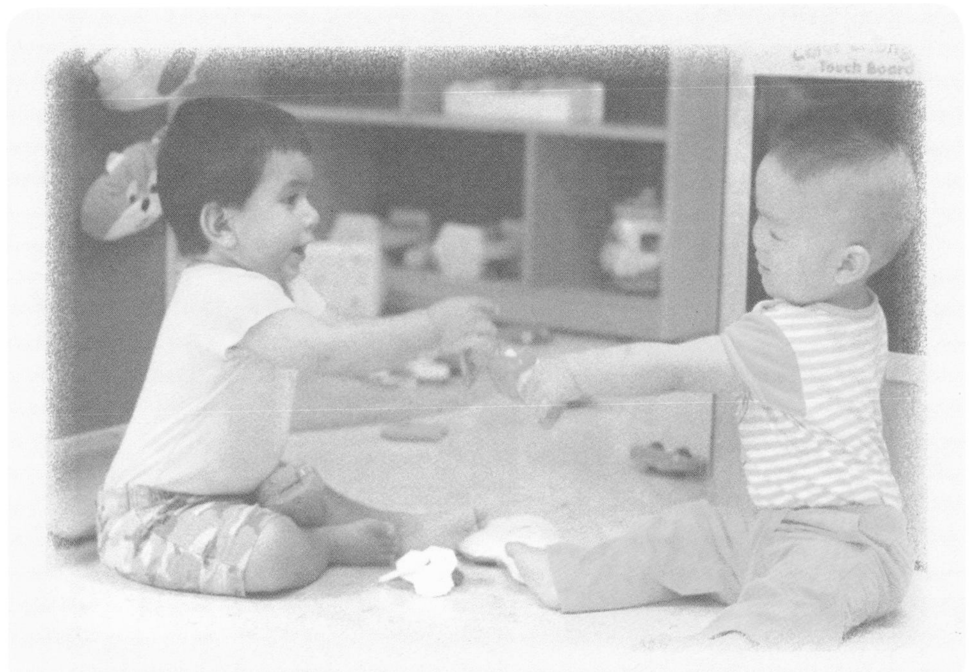
Touch Board

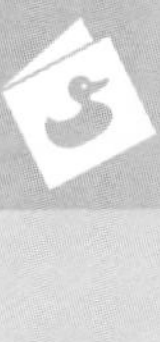

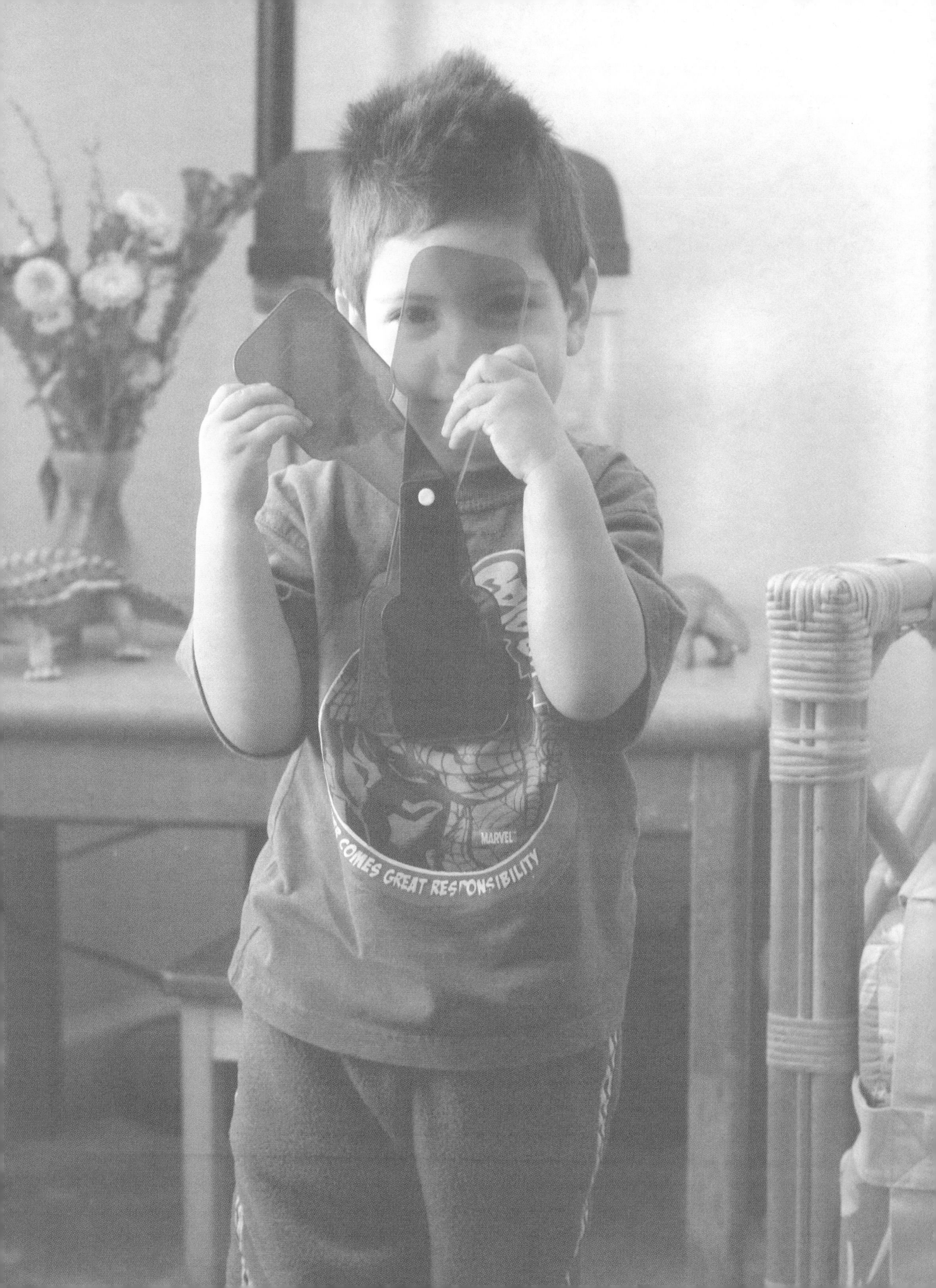
MARVEL
COMES GREAT RESPONSIBILITY

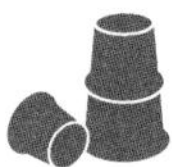

Cognitive Development

"The last two decades of infancy research have seen dramatic changes in the way developmental psychologists characterize the earliest stages of cognitive development. The infant, once regarded as an organism driven mainly by simple sensorimotor schemes, is now seen as possessing sophisticated cognitive skills and even sophisticated concepts that guide knowledge acquisition" (Madole and Oakes 1999, 263).

"What we see in the crib is the greatest mind that has ever existed, the most powerful learning machine in the universe" (Gopnik, Meltzoff, and Kuhl 1999, 1).

The term *cognitive development* refers to the process of growth and change in intellectual/mental abilities such as thinking, reasoning and understanding. It includes the acquisition and consolidation of knowledge. Infants draw on social-emotional, language, motor, and perceptual experiences and abilities for cognitive development. They are attuned to relationships between features of objects, actions, and the physical environment. But they are particularly attuned to people. Parents, family members, friends, teachers, and caregivers play a vital role in supporting the cognitive development of infants by providing the healthy interpersonal or social-emotional context in which cognitive development unfolds. Caring, responsive adults provide the base from which infants can fully engage in behaviors and interactions that promote learning. Such adults also serve as a prime source of imitation.

Cultural context is important to young children's cognitive development. There is substantial variation in how intelligence is defined within different cultures (Sternberg and Grigorenko 2004). As a result, different aspects of cognitive functioning or cognitive performance may be more highly valued in some cultural contexts than in others. For example, whereas processing speed is an aspect of intelligence that is highly valued within the predominant Western conceptualizations of intelligence, "Ugandan villagers associate intelligence with adjectives such as *slow, careful,* and *active*" (Rogoff and Chavajay 1995, 865.). Aspects of intelligence that have to do with social competence appear to be seen as more important than speed

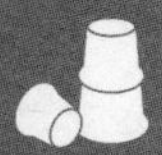

in some non-Western cultural contexts (Sternberg and Grigorenko 2004). Certainly, it is crucial for early childhood professionals to recognize the role that cultural context plays in defining and setting the stage for children's healthy cognitive functioning.

Research has identified a broad range of cognitive competencies and described the remarkable progression of cognitive development during the early childhood years. Experts in the field describe infants as active, motivated, and engaged learners who possess an impressive range of cognitive competencies (National Research Council and Institute of Medicine 2000) and learn through exploration (Whitehurst and Lonigan 1998). Infants demonstrate natural curiosity. They have a strong drive to learn and act accordingly. In fact, they have been described as "born to learn" (National Research Council and Institute of Medicine 2000, 148).

Cause-and-Effect

Everyday experiences—for example, crying and then being picked up or waving a toy and then hearing it rattle—provide opportunities for infants to learn about cause and effect. "Even very young infants possess expectations about physical events" (Baillargeon 2004, 89). This knowledge helps infants better understand the properties of objects, the patterns of human behavior, and the relationship between events and the consequences. Through developing an understanding of cause and effect, infants build their abilities to solve problems, to make predictions, and to understand the impact of their behavior on others.

Spatial Relationships

Infants learn about spatial relationships in a variety of ways; for example, exploring objects with their mouths, tracking objects and people visually, squeezing into tight spaces, fitting objects into openings, and looking at things from different perspectives (Mangione, Lally, and Signer 1992). They spend much of their time exploring the physical and spatial aspects of the environment, including the characteristics of, and interrelationships between, the people, objects, and the physical space around them (Clements 2004). The development of an understanding of spatial relationships increases infants' knowledge of how things move and fit in space and the properties of objects (their bodies and the physical environment).

Problem Solving

Infants exhibit a high level of interest in solving problems. Even very young infants will work to solve a problem, for example, how to find their fingers in order to suck on them (National Research Council and Institute of Medicine 2000). Older infants may solve the problem of how to reach an interesting toy that is out of reach by trying to roll toward it or by gesturing to an adult for help. Infants and toddlers solve problems by varied means, including physically acting on objects, using learning schemes they have developed, imitating solutions found by others, using objects or other people as tools, and using trial and error.

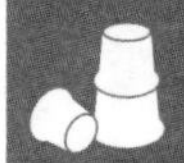

Imitation

Imitation is broadly understood to be a powerful way to learn. It has been identified as crucial in the acquisition of cultural knowledge (Rogoff 1990) and language. Imitation by newborns has been demonstrated for adult facial expressions (Meltzoff and Moore 1983), head movements, and tongue protrusions (Meltzoff and Moore 1989). "The findings of imitation in human newborns highlighted predispositions to imitate facial and manual actions, vocalizations and emotionally laden facial expressions" (Bard and Russell 1999, 93). Infant imitation involves perception and motor processes (Meltzoff and Moore 1999). The very early capacity to imitate makes possible imitation games in which the adult mirrors the child's behavior, such as sticking out one's tongue or matching the pitch of a sound the infant makes, and then the infant imitates back. This type of interaction builds over time as the infant and the adult add elements and variations in their imitation games.

Infants engage in both immediate imitation and delayed imitation. Immediate imitation occurs when infants observe and immediately attempt to copy or mimic behavior. For example, immediate imitation can be seen when an infant's parent sticks out his tongue and the infant sticks out his tongue in response. As infants develop, they are able to engage in delayed imitation, repeating the behavior of others at a later time after having observed it. An example of delayed imitation is a child reenacting part of a parent's exercise routine, such as lifting a block several times as if it were a weight. Butterworth (1999, 63) sums up the importance of early imitation in the following manner: "Modern research has shown imitation to be a natural mechanism of learning and communication which deserves to be at centre stage in developmental psychology."

Memory

The capacity to remember allows infants and toddlers to differentiate between familiar and unfamiliar people and objects, anticipate and participate in parts of personal care routines, learn language, and come to know the rules of social interaction. The infant's memory system is quite remarkable and functions at a higher level than was previously believed (Howe and Courage 1993). Although age is not the only determinant of memory functioning, as infants get older they are able to retain information for longer periods of time (Bauer 2004). Infants exhibit long-term recall well before they are able to articulate their past experiences verbally (Bauer 2002b).

The emergence of memory is related to the development of a neural network with various components (Bauer 2002b). Commenting on the different forms and functions of early memory development, Bauer (2002a, 131) states: "It is widely believed that memory is not a unitary trait but is comprised of different systems or processes, which serve distinct functions, and are characterized by fundamentally different rules of operation." Bauer (2002a, 145) later adds that recent research counters earlier suggestions that preschool-aged children demonstrate little memory capacity and to speculations that younger children and infants demonstrate little or no memory capacity. Bauer (2002a,

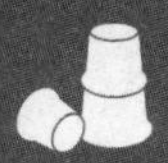

145) concludes: "It is now clear that from early in life, the human organism stores information over the long term and that the effects of prior experience are apparent in behavior. In the first months of life, infants exhibit recognition memory for all manner of natural and artificial stimuli."

Number Sense

Number sense refers to children's concepts of numbers and the relationships among number concepts. Research findings indicate that infants as young as five months of age are sensitive to number and are able to discriminate among small sets of up to three objects (Starkey and Cooper 1980; Starkey, Spelke, and Gelman 1990). Infants demonstrate the ability to quickly and accurately recognize the quantity in a small set of objects without counting. This ability is called subitizing.

According to one theoretical perspective, infants' abilities to discriminate among numbers, for example, two versus three objects, does not reflect "number knowledge." Rather, this early skill appears to be based on infants' perceptual abilities to "see" small arrangements of number (Clements 2004; Carey 2001), or on their ability to notice a change in the general amount of objects they are seeing (Mix, Huttenlocher, and Levine 2002). The alternative view is that the infant's early sensitivity to number is numerical in nature. In other words, infants have a capacity to distinguish among numbers and to reason about these numbers in numerically meaningful ways (Wynn 1998; Gallistel and Gelman 1992). In some sense, they know that three objects are more than one object. Whether early number sensitivity is solely perceptual in nature or also numerical in nature, developmental theorists agree that it sets the foundation for the later development of children's understanding of number and quantity.

As children's understanding and use of language increases, they begin to assimilate language based on number knowledge to their nonverbal knowledge of number and quantity (Baroody 2004). Between 18 and 24 months of age, children use relational words to indicate "more" or "same" as well as number words. They begin to count aloud, typically starting with "one" and continuing with a stream of number names (Fuson 1988; Gelman and Gallistel 1978), although they may omit some numbers and not use the conventional number list (e.g. "one, two, three, seven, nine, ten"). Around the same age, children also begin to count small collections of objects; however, they may point to the same item twice or say a number word without pointing to an object. And they begin to construct an understanding of cardinality (i.e., the last number word is used when counting represents the total number of objects).

Classification

Classification refers to the infant's developing ability to group, sort, categorize, connect, and have expectations of objects and people according to their attributes. Three-month-olds demonstrate that they expect people to act differently than objects (Legerstee 1997). They also demonstrate the ability to discriminate between smiling and frowning expressions (Barrera and Maurer 1981). Mandler (2000)

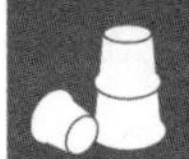

distinguishes between two types of categorization made by infants: perceptual and conceptual. Perceptual categorization has to do with similarities or differences infants sense, such as similarities in visual appearance. Conceptual categorization has to do with grouping based on what objects do or how they act. According to Mareschal and French (2000, 59), "the ability to categorize underlies much of cognition." Classification is a fundamental skill in both problem solving and symbolic play.

Symbolic Play

Symbolic play is a common early childhood behavior also called "pretend play, make-believe play, fantasy play . . . or imaginative play" (Gowen 1995, 75). Representational thinking is a core component of symbolic play. At around eight months of age, infants have learned the functions of common objects (for example, holding a play telephone to "hear" Grandma's voice). By the time children are around 18 months of age, they use one object to stand for, or represent, another. For example, an 18-month-old may pretend a banana is a telephone. At around 36 months, children engage in make-believe play in which they represent an object without having that object, or a concrete substitute, available. For example, they may make a "phone call" by holding their hand up to their ear.

As children approach 36 months of age, they increasingly engage in pretend play in which they reenact familiar events. Make-believe play allows older infants to try to better understand social roles, engage in communication with others, and revisit and make sense of past experiences. Research suggests that engaging in pretend play appears to be related to young children's developing understanding of other people's feelings and beliefs (Youngblade and Dunn 1995). Outdoor environments, such as sandboxes (Moser 1995) or play structures, offer rich opportunities for symbolic play or pretending. Although outdoor play areas are often considered most in terms of motor behavior or physical activity, they also offer special opportunities for symbolic play (Perry 2003). For example, children playing outside may pretend to garden or may use a large wheeled toy to reenact going on a shopping trip.

Attention Maintenance

Attention maintenance has been described as a form of cognitive self-regulation. It refers to the infant's growing ability to exercise control over his attention or concentration (Bronson 2000). Attention maintenance permits infants to gather information, to sustain learning experiences, to observe, and to problem-solve. Infants demonstrate attention maintenance when they attend to people, actions, and things they find interesting even in the presence of distractions. The ability to maintain attention/concentration is an important self-regulatory skill related to learning. There is significant variability in attentiveness even among typically developing children (Ruff and Rothbart 1996).

Understanding of Personal Care Routines

Personal care activities are a routine part of the young child's daily life. They also present significant opportu-

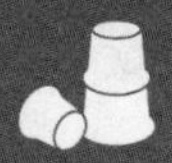

nities for learning in both child care settings and at home. Infants' growing abilities to anticipate, understand, and participate in these routines represent a significant aspect of their cognitive functioning, one related to their abilities to understand their relationships with others, their abilities to take care of themselves, and their skills in group participation. At first, young infants respond to the adult's actions during these routines. Then they begin to participate more actively (O'Brien 1997). Understanding the steps involved in personal care routines and anticipating next steps are skills related to the cognitive foundations of attention maintenance, imitation, memory, cause-and-effect, and problem solving. The cultural perspectives of the adults who care for infants are related to their expectations for the degree of independence or self-initiation children demonstrate during personal care routines. Depending on their cultural experiences, children may vary greatly in their understanding of personal care routines.

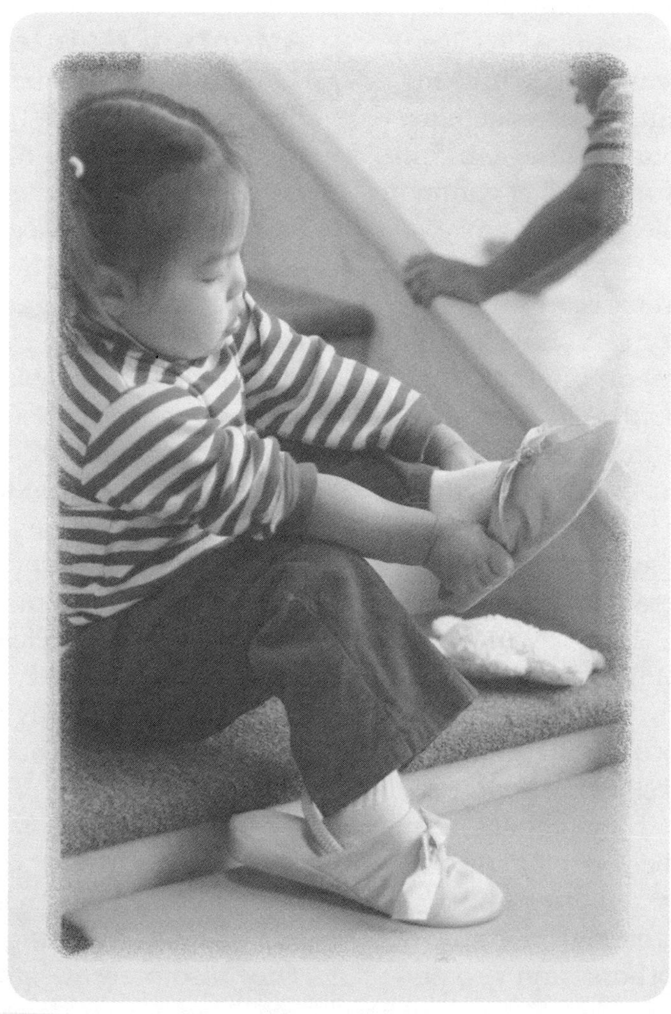

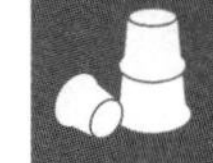

Foundation: Cause-and-Effect

The developing understanding that one event brings about another

8 months	*18 months*	*36 months*
At around eight months of age, children perform simple actions to make things happen, notice the relationships between events, and notice the effects of others on the immediate environment.	At around 18 months of age, children combine simple actions to cause things to happen or change the way they interact with objects and people in order to see how it changes the outcome.	At around 36 months of age, children demonstrate an understanding of cause and effect by making predictions about what could happen and reflect upon what caused something to happen. (California Department of Education [CDE] 2005)
For example, the child may:	**For example, the child may:**	**For example, the child may:**
• Shake a toy, hear the sound it makes, and then shake it again. (5.5–8 mos.; Parks 2004, 58) • Loudly bang a spoon on the table, notice the loud sound, and do it again. (By 7 mos.; American Academy of Pediatrics 2004, 210; 8 mos.; Meisels and others 2003, 21) • Watch the infant care teacher wind up a music box and, when the music stops, touch her hand to get her to make it start again. (5–9 mos.; Parks 2004, 58) • Splash hands in water and notice how his face gets wet. (4–10 mos.; Ginsburg and Opper 1988, 43) • Push a button on the push-button toy and watch the figure pop up. (6–9 mos.; Lerner and Ciervo 2003) • Put objects into a clear container, turn it over and watch the objects fall out, and then fill it up again. (8 mos.; Meisels and others 2003, 21) • Clap hands and then look at a parent to get her to play pat-a-cake. (8 mos.; Meisels and others 2003, 21)	• Try to wind the handle of a pop-up toy after not being able to open the top. (15 mos.; Brazelton 1992, 161) • Drop different objects from various heights to see how they fall and to hear the noise they make when they land. (12–18 mos.; Ginsburg and Opper 1988, 56) • Build a tower with the big cardboard blocks and kick it over to make it fall, then build it again and knock it down with a hand. (18 mos.; Meisels and others 2003, 37) • Use a wooden spoon to bang on different pots and pans, and notice how the infant care teacher responds when the child hits the pans harder and makes a louder noise. (18 mos.; Meisels and others 2003, 37)	• Communicate, "She misses her mommy" when a child cries after her mother leaves in the morning. • Make a prediction about what will happen next in the story when the infant care teacher asks, "What do you think will happen next?" • Answer the infant care teacher when she asks, "What do you think your mom's going to say when you give her your picture?" • See a bandage on a peer's knee and ask, "What happened?" • Push the big green button to make the tape recorder play. (By 36 mos.; American Academy of Pediatrics 2004, 308) • Walk quietly when the baby is sleeping.

Chart continues on next page.

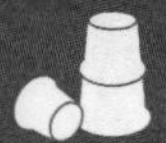

Cause-and-Effect

Behaviors leading up to the foundation (4 to 7 months)	Behaviors leading up to the foundation (9 to 17 months)	Behaviors leading up to the foundation (19 to 35 months)
During this period, the child may: • Hear a loud noise and turn head in the direction of the noise. (3.5–5 mos.; Parks 2004, 37) • Explore toys with hands and mouth. (3–6 mos.; Parks 2004, 10) • Move body in a rocking motion to get the infant care teacher to continue rocking. (4–5 mos.; Parks 2004, 57; Birth–8 mos.; Lerner and Dombro 2000) • Kick legs in the crib and notice that the mobile up above jiggles with the kicking movements. (4–5 mos.; American Academy of Pediatrics 2004, 209) • Attend to a toy while exploring it with the hands. (Scaled score of 9 for 5:16–6:15 mos.; Bayley 2006, 55)	During this period, the child may: • Hold a block in each hand and bang the blocks together. (8.5–12 mos.; Parks 2004) • Keep turning an object around to find the side that makes it work, such as the reflective side of a mirror, or the open side of a nesting cup. (9–12 mos.; Parks 2004, 65) • Cry and anticipate that the infant care teacher will come to help. (9–12 mos.; Lerner and Ciervo 2003) • Drop an object repeatedly from the chair to hear it clang on the floor or to get the infant care teacher to come pick it up. (9–12 mos.; Parks 2004, 65) • Watch the infant care teacher squeeze the toy in the water table to make water squirt out, then try the same action. (Scaled score of 10 for 13:16–14:15 mos.; Bayley 2006, 61) • Hand a toy car to a family member after it stops moving and the child cannot figure out how to make it move again. (12–15 mos.; Parks 2004, 59) • Close eyes and turn face away from the water table before splashing with hands. (12 mos.; Meisels and others 2003, 28) • Continue to push the button on a toy that is broken and appear confused or frustrated when nothing happens. (12 mos.; Meisels and others 2003, 29)	During this period, the child may: • Roll cars of different sizes down the slide. (18–24 mos.; Lerner and Ciervo 2003)

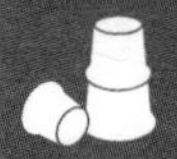

Foundation: Spatial Relationships

The developing understanding of how things move and fit in space

8 months	*18 months*	*36 months*
At around eight months of age, children move their bodies, explore the size and shape of objects, and observe people and objects as they move through space.	At around 18 months of age, children use trial and error to discover how things move and fit in space. (12–18 mos.; Parks 2004, 81)	At around 36 months of age, children can predict how things will fit and move in space without having to try out every possible solution, and show understanding of words used to describe size and locations in space.
For example, the child may:	**For example, the child may:**	**For example, the child may:**
• Use vision or hearing to track the path of someone walking by. (5.5–8 mos.; Parks 2004, 64; birth–8 mos.; Lally and others 1995, 78–79) • Watch a ball roll away after accidentally knocking it. (5.5–8 mos., Parks 2004, 64) • Hold one stacking cup in each hand. (6.5–7.5 mos.; Parks 2004, 50) • Put toys into a clear container, dump them out, and then fill the container up again. (8 mos.; Meisels and others 2003, 21)	• Go around the back of a chair to get the toy car that rolled behind it instead of trying to follow the car's path by squeezing underneath the chair. (12–18 mos.; Parks 2004 67; 8–18 mos.; Lally and others 1995, 78–79) • Use two hands to pick up a big truck, but only one hand to pick up a small one. (12–18 mos.; Parks 2004, 81) • Put a smaller nesting cup inside a larger cup after trying it the other way around. (12–18 mos.; Parks 2004, 81) • Choose a large cookie off the plate instead of a smaller one. (12–18 mos.; Parks 2004, 81) • Put the child-sized hat on his head and the larger hat on the infant care teacher's head. (12–18 mos.; Parks 2004, 81) • Stack three nesting cups inside one another, after trying some combinations that do not work. (12–19 mos.; Parks 2004, 82) • Put one or two pegs into the pegboard. (14:16–15:15 mos.; Bayley 2006, 62) • Roll a ball back and forth with the infant care teacher. (18 mos.; Meisels and others 2003, 38) • Fit pieces into a puzzle board. (18 mos.; Meisels and others 2003, 39) • Try to fit a piece into the shape sorter and, when it does not fit, turn it until it fits. (12–19 mos.; Parks 2004, 82)	• Hand the big truck to a peer who asks for the big one. (Scaled score of 10 for 28:16–30:15 mos.; Bayley 2006, 95) • Use words such as *big* and *little.* (25–30 mos.; Parks 2004, 82; 36 mos.; Meisels and others 2003, 73) • Put together a puzzle with three to four separate pieces. (By 36 mos.; American Academy of Pediatrics 2004, 308; 30–36 mos.; Parks 2004, 68) • Get the serving spoon off the tray when the infant care teacher asks for the big spoon, even though there are small spoons on the tray. (30–36 mos.; Parks 2004, 83) • Stack rings onto a post with the biggest ring on the bottom and the smallest ring on the top, without much trial and error. (30–36 mos.; Parks 2004, 83; 24–36 mos.; *Engaging Young Children* 2004, 44) • Point to a peer's stick when the infant care teacher asks which stick is longer. (33–36 mos.; Parks 2004, 83; 24–36 mos.; *Engaging Young Children* 2004, 53) • Understand requests that include simple prepositions; for example, "Please put your cup on the table" or "Please get your blanket out of your back pack." (By 36 mos.; Coplan 1993, 2; by 36 mos.; American Academy of Pediatrics 2004; 24–36 mos.; *Engaging Young Children* 2004) • Move around an obstacle when going from one place to another. (24–36 mos.; American Academy of Pediatrics 2004, 303)

Chart continues on next page.

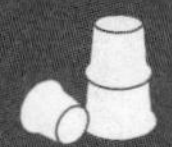

Spatial Relationships

Behaviors leading up to the foundation (4 to 7 months)	Behaviors leading up to the foundation (9 to 17 months)	Behaviors leading up to the foundation (19 to 35 months)
During this period, the child may: • Look at her own hand. (Scaled score of 9 for 4:06–4:15 mos.; Bayley 2006, 53) • Reach for a nearby toy and try to grasp it. (4.5–5.5 mos.; Parks 2004; scaled score of 10 for 4:16–4:25 mos.; Bayley 2006, 54) • Explore toys with hands and mouth. (3–6 mos.; Parks 2004, 10)	During this period, the child may: • Roll a car back and forth on the floor. (6–11 mos.; Parks 2004, 26) • Dump toys out of a container. (9–11 mos.; Parks 2004, 64) • Turn a toy to explore all sides to figure out how it works. (9–12 mos.; Parks 2004, 65) • Throw or drop a spoon or cup from the table and watch as it falls. (9–12 mos.; Parks 2004, 65) • Take rings off a stacking ring toy. (10–11 mos.; Parks 2004, 65) • Move over and between cushions and pillows on the floor. (8–12 mos.; American Academy of Pediatrics 2004, 234) • Crawl down a few carpeted stairs. (Around 12 mos.; American Academy of Pediatrics 2004, 234) • See a ball roll under the couch and then reach under the couch. (12–13 mos.; Parks 2004, 66) • Stack one block on top of another one. (12–16 mos.; Parks 2004, 66) • Put one or two rings back onto the post of a stacking ring toy. (13–15 mos.; Parks 2004, 66) • Put the circle piece of a puzzle into the round opening, after trying the triangle opening and the square opening. (Scaled score of 10 for 15:16–16:15 mos.; Bayley 2006, 63)	During this period, the child may: • Complete a puzzle of three separate cut-out pieces, such as a circle, square, and triangle. (Scaled score of 10 for 19:16–20:15 mos.; Bayley 2006, 66) • Fit many pegs into a pegboard. (Scaled score of 10 for 21:16–22:15 mos.; Bayley 2006, 68) • Turn a book right-side up after realizing that it is upside down. (18–24 mos.; Parks 2004) • Fit four nesting cups in the correct order, even if it takes a couple of tries. (19–24 mos.; Parks 2004, 82) • Assemble a two-piece puzzle; for example, a picture of a flower cut into two pieces. (Scaled score of 10 for 23:16–24:15 mos.; Bayley 2006, 69)

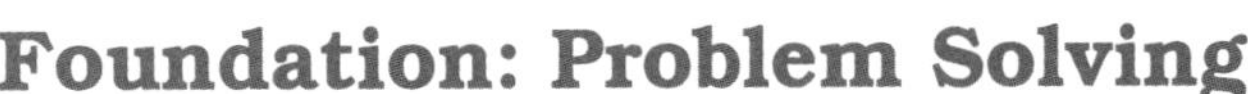

Foundation: Problem Solving

The developing ability to engage in a purposeful effort to reach a goal or figure out how something works

8 months	*18 months*	*36 months*
At around eight months of age, children use simple actions to try to solve problems involving objects, their bodies, or other people.	At around 18 months of age, children use a number of ways to solve problems: physically trying out possible solutions before finding one that works; using objects as tools; watching someone else solve the problem and then applying the same solution; or gesturing or vocalizing to someone else for help.	At around 36 months of age, children solve some problems without having to physically try out every possible solution and may ask for help when needed. (By 36 mos.; American Academy of Pediatrics 2004, 308)
For example, the child may:	**For example, the child may:**	**For example, the child may:**
• Shake, bang, and squeeze toys repeatedly to make the sounds happen again and again. (5.5–8 mos.; Parks 2004, 58; by 12 mos.; American Academy of Pediatrics 2004, 243) • Reach for a ball as it rolls away. (5.5–8 mos.; Parks 2004, 64) • Vocalize to get the infant care teacher's attention. (6.5–8 mos.; Parks 2004) • Pull the string on a toy to make it come closer. (8 mos.; Meisels and others 2003, 21) • Focus on a desired toy that is just out of reach while repeatedly reaching for it. (5–9 mos.; Parks 2004, 49) • Turn the bottle over to get the nipple in his mouth. • Lift up a scarf to search for a toy that is hidden underneath. (By 8 mos.; American Academy of Pediatrics 2004, 244)	• Pull the string of a pull toy to get it closer even when the toy gets momentarily stuck on something. (18 mos.; Meisels and others 2003, 38) • Use the handle of a toy broom to dislodge a ball under the bookshelf. (8–18 mos.; Lally and others 1995, 78–79) • Bring a small stool over to reach a toy on top of a shelf, having observed the infant care teacher do it. (8–18 mos.; Lally and others 1995, 78–79) • Look at a plate of crackers that is out of reach and then at the infant care teacher, and communicate "more." (Scaled score of 10 for 16:16–17:15 mos.; Bayley 2006; 14–20 mos.; Parks 2004) • Hand the infant care teacher a puzzle piece that the child is having trouble with.	• Ignore the stick that is much too short to reach a desired object and choose a stick that looks as if it may be long enough. • Stack only the cubes with holes in them on the stacking post, ignoring the cube-shaped blocks without holes that got mixed into the bin. (18–36 mos.; Lally and others 1995, 78–79) • Place the triangle piece into the puzzle without first needing to try it in the round or square hole. (By 36 mos.; American Academy of Pediatrics 2004, 306) • Ask the infant care teacher for help with the lid of a jar of paint. (36 mos.; Meisels and others 2003, 75) • Ask a peer to help move the train tracks over so that the child can build a block tower on the floor. (36 mos.; Meisels and others 2003, 75) • Ask or gesture for the infant care teacher to help tie the child's shoelace. (36 mos.; Meisels and others 2003, 75)

Chart continues on next page.

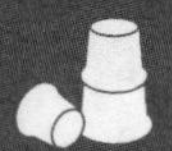

Problem Solving

Behaviors leading up to the foundation (4 to 7 months)	Behaviors leading up to the foundation (9 to 17 months)	Behaviors leading up to the foundation (19 to 35 months)
During this period, the child may: • Explore toys with hands and mouth. (3–6 mos.; Parks 2004, 10) • Reach for a second toy when already holding on to one toy. (5–6.5 mos.; Parks 2004, 49) • Hold a toy up to look at it while exploring it with the hands. (Scaled score of 9 for 5:16–6:15 mos.; Bayley 2006, 55)	During this period, the child may: • Crawl over a pile of soft blocks to get to the big red ball. (8–11 mos.; Parks 2004) • Figure out how toys work by repeating the same actions over and over again. (9–12 mos.; Lerner and Ciervo 2003) • Pull the blanket in order to obtain the toy that is lying out of reach on top of the blanket. (8–10 mos.; Parks 2004) • Crawl around the legs of a chair to get to the ball that rolled behind it. (9–12 mos.; Parks 2004, 50; 18 mos.; Lally and others 1995, 78–79) • Keep turning an object around to find the side that makes it work, such as the reflective side of a mirror or the open side of a nesting cup. (9–12 mos.; Parks 2004, 65) • Try to hold on to two toys with one hand while reaching for a third desired toy, even if not successful. (Scaled score of 9 for 10:16–11:15 mos.; Bayley 2006, 58) • Unscrew the lid of a plastic jar to get items out of it. (Scaled score of 10 for 14:16–15:15 mos.; Bayley 2006, 62)	During this period, the child may: • Use a stick to dig in the sandbox when unable to find a shovel. (17–24 mos.; Parks 2004) • Use a tool to solve a problem, such as using the toy broom to get a car out from under the couch, using a wooden puzzle base as a tray to carry all the puzzle pieces to another place, or using the toy shopping cart to pick up the wooden blocks and move them to the shelf to be put away. (17–24 mos.; Parks 2004, 52) • Move to the door and try to turn the knob after a parent leaves for work in the morning. (21–23 mos.; Parks 2004, 53) • Imitate a problem-solving method that the child has observed someone else do before. (Scaled score of 10 for 20:16–21:15 mos.; Bayley 2006, 66) • Tug on shoelaces in order to untie them. • Complete a puzzle with three separate cut-out pieces, such as a circle, square, and triangle, even though the child may try to put the triangle into the square hole before fitting it in the triangle opening. (Scaled score of 10 for 19:16–20:15 mos.; Bayley 2006, 66)

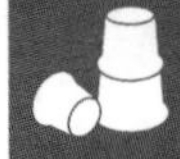

Foundation: Imitation

The developing ability to mirror, repeat, and practice the actions of others, either immediately or later

8 months	*18 months*	*36 months*
At around 8 months of age, children imitate simple actions and expressions of others during interactions.	At around 18 months of age, children imitate others' actions that have more than one step and imitate simple actions that they have observed others doing at an earlier time. (Parks 2004; 28)	At around 36 months of age, children reenact multiple steps of others' actions that they have observed at an earlier time. (30–36 mos.; Parks 2004, 29)
For example, the child may:	**For example, the child may:**	**For example, the child may:**
• Copy the infant care teacher's movements when playing pat-a-cake and peek-a-boo. (Coplan 1993, 3) • Imitate a familiar gesture, such as clapping hands together or patting a doll's back, after seeing the infant care teacher do it. (7–8 mos.; Parks 2004) • Notice how the infant care teacher makes a toy work and then push the same button to make it happen again. (6–9 mos.; Lerner and Ciervo 2003)	• Imitate simple actions that she has observed adults doing; for example, take a toy phone out of a purse and say hello as a parent does. (12–18 mos.; Lerner and Ciervo 2003) • Pretend to sweep with a child-sized broom, just as a family member does at home. (15–18 mos.; Parks 2004, 27) • Rock the baby doll to sleep, just as a parent does with the new baby. (15–18 mos.; Parks 2004, 27) • Imitate using the toy hammer as a parent did. (18 mos.; Meisels and others 2003, 38)	• Reenact the steps of a family celebration that the child attended last weekend. (29–36 mos.; Hart and Risley 1999, 118–19) • Pretend to get ready for work or school by making breakfast, packing lunch, grabbing a purse, and communicating good-bye before heading out the door. (30–36 mos.; Parks 2004, 29)

Chart continues on next page.

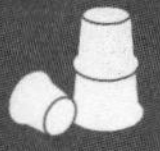

Imitation

Behaviors leading up to the foundation (4 to 7 months)	Behaviors leading up to the foundation (9 to 17 months)	Behaviors leading up to the foundation (19 to 35 months)
During this period, the child may: • Listen to the infant care teacher talk during a diaper change and then babble back when she pauses. (5.5–6.5 mos.; Parks 2004, 125) • Copy the intonation of the infant care teacher's speech when babbling. (7 mos.; Parks 2004)	During this period, the child may: • Shrug shoulders after the infant care teacher does it. (9–11 mos.; Parks 2004; by 12 mos.; American Academy of Pediatrics 2004, 243) • Imitate sounds or words immediately after the infant care teacher makes them. (9 mos.; Apfel and Provence 2001; 12–18 mos.; Hulit and Howard 2006, 122; 17 mos.; Hart and Risley 1999, 84) • Copy the infant care teacher in waving "bye-bye" to a parent as he leaves the room. (12 mos.; Meisels and others 2003, 26) • Copy an adult's action that is unfamiliar but that the child can see herself do, such as wiggling toes, even though it may take some practice before doing it exactly as the adult does. (9–14 mos.; Parks 2004, 32) • Watch the infant care teacher squeeze the toy in the water table to make water squirt out, then try the same action. (Scaled score of 10 for 13:16–14:15 mos.; Bayley 2006, 61) • Imitate the hand motion of the infant care teacher. (Scaled score of 10 for 14:16–15:15 mos.; Bayley 2006, 135) • Point to or indicate an object, pay attention as the infant care teacher labels the object, and then try to repeat the label. (11–16 mos.; Hart and Risley 1999, 82)	During this period, the child may: • Repeat the most important word of a sentence the infant care teacher has just communicated. (17–19 mos.; Parks 2004) • Imitate the last word or last few words of what an adult just said; for example say, cup or a cup after the infant care teacher says, "That's a cup" or say, "Daddy bye-bye" after the mother says, "Daddy went bye-bye." (22 mos.; Hart and Risley 1999, 99; 17–19 mos.; Parks 2004, 128) • Copy several actions that the child cannot see himself doing, such as wrinkling the nose. (17–20 mos.; Parks 2004, 32) • Say, "beep, beep, beep, beep" after hearing the garbage truck back up outside. (18-21 mos.; Parks 2004) • Act out a few steps of a familiar routine, such as pretend to fill the tub, bathe a baby doll, and dry the doll. (18–24 mos.; Parks 2004, 28) • Imitate words that the adult has expressed to the child at an earlier time, not immediately after hearing them. (24–27 mos.; Parks 2004; 19–28 mos.; Hart and Risley 1999, 61) • Imitate two new actions of the infant care teacher; for example, put one hand on head and point with the other hand. (26:16–27:15 mos.; Bayley 2006, 71) • Imitate the way a family member communicates by using the same gestures, unique words, and intonation.

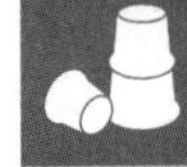

Foundation: Memory

The developing ability to store and later retrieve information about past experiences

8 months	*18 months*	*36 months*
At around 8 months of age, children recognize familiar people, objects, and routines in the environment and show awareness that familiar people still exist even when they are no longer physically present.	At around 18 months of age, children remember typical actions of people, the location of objects, and steps of routines.	At around 36 months of age, children anticipate the series of steps in familiar activities, events, or routines; remember characteristics of the environment or people in it; and may briefly describe recent past events or act them out. (24–36 mos.; Seigel 1999, 33)
For example, the child may:	**For example, the child may:**	**For example, the child may:**
• Turn toward the front door when hearing the doorbell ring or toward the phone when hearing the phone ring. (8 mos.; Meisels and others 2003, 20) • Look for the father after he briefly steps out of the child care room during drop-off in the morning. (8 mos.; Meisels and others 2003, 20)	• Get a blanket from the doll cradle because that is where baby blankets are usually stored, after the infant care teacher says, "The baby is tired. Where's her blanket?" (15–18 mos.; Parks 2004, 67) • Anticipate and participate in the steps of a nap routine. (18 mos.; Fogel 2001, 368) • Watch the infant care teacher placing a toy inside one of three pots with lids and reach for the correct lid when the teacher asks where the toy went. (8–18 mos.; Lally and others 1995, 78–79) • Continue to search for an object even though it is hidden under something distracting, such as a soft blanket or a crinkly piece of paper. • See a photo of a close family member and say his name or hug the photo. • Go to the cubby to get his blanket that is inside the diaper bag.	• Communicate, "Big slide" after a trip to neighborhood park. (24–36 mos.; Seigel 1999, 33) • Tell a parent, "Today we jumped in the puddles" when picked up from school. (Siegel 1999, 34) • Recall an event in the past, such as the time a family member came to school and made a snack. (18–36 mos.; Siegel 1999, 46) • Identify which child is absent from school that day by looking around the snack table and figuring out who is missing. (18–36 mos.; Lally and others 1995, 78–79) • Act out a trip to the grocery store by getting a cart, putting food in it, and paying for the food. (24 mos.; Bauer and Mandler 1989) • Get her pillow out of the cubby, in anticipation of naptime as soon as lunch is finished.

Chart continues on next page.

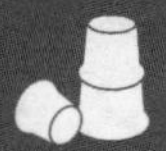

Memory

Behaviors leading up to the foundation (4 to 7 months)	Behaviors leading up to the foundation (9 to 17 months)	Behaviors leading up to the foundation (19 to 35 months)
During this period, the child may: • Explore toys with hands and mouth. (3–6 mos.; Parks 2004, 10) • Find a rattle hidden under a blanket when only the handle is showing. (4–6 mos.; Parks 2004, 42) • Look toward the floor when the bottle falls off table. (Scaled score of 10 for 5:06–5:15 mos.; Bayley 2006, 55; 8 mos.; Meisels and others 2003, 20; birth–8 mos.; Lally and others 1995, 72)	During this period, the child may: • Ask for a parent after morning drop-off. (9–12 mos.; Lerner and Ciervo 2003) • Reach in the infant care teacher's pocket after watching him hide a toy there. (11–13 mos.; Parks 2004, 43) • Look or reach inside a container of small toys after seeing the infant care teacher take the toys off the table and put them in the container. (Scaled score of 10 for 8:16–9:15 mos.; Bayley 2006, 57; birth–8 mos.; Lally and others 1995, 78–79) • Lift a scarf to search for a toy after seeing the infant care teacher hide it under the scarf. (By 8 mos.; American Academy of Pediatrics 2004, 244; 8 mos.; Kail 1990, 112)	During this period, the child may: • Say "meow" when the infant care teacher points to the picture of the cat and asks what the cat says. (12–24 mos.; Siegel 1999, 32) • Give another child an object that belongs to her. (12–24 mos.; Siegel 1999, 32) • Remember where toys should be put away in the classroom. (21–24 mos.; Parks 2004, 318) • Find a hidden toy, even when it is hidden under two or three blankets. (By 24 mos.; American Academy of Pediatrics 2004, 273) • Express "mama" when the infant care teacher asks who packed the child's snack.

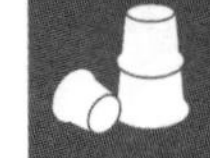

Foundation: Number Sense

The developing understanding of number and quantity

8 months	*18 months*	*36 months*
At around eight months of age, children usually focus on one object or person at a time, yet they may at times hold two objects, one in each hand.	At around 18 months of age, children demonstrate understanding that there are different amounts of things.	At around 36 months of age, children show some understanding that numbers represent how many and demonstrate understanding of words that identify how much. (By 36 mos.; American Academy of Pediatrics 2004, 308)
For example, the child may:	**For example, the child may:**	**For example, the child may:**
• Hold one block in each hand, then drop one of them when the infant care teacher holds out a third block for the child to hold. (6.5–7.5 mos.; Parks 2004, 50) • Watch a ball as it rolls away after hitting it with her hand. (5.5–8 mos.; Parks 2004, 64) • Explore one toy at a time by shaking, banging, or squeezing it. (5.5–8 mos:; Parks 2004, 58; 8 mos.; Meisels and others 2003, 21; birth–8 mos.; Lally and others 1995, 78–79) • Notice when someone walks in the room.	• Communicate "more" and point to a bowl of apple slices. (18 mos.; Meisels and others 2003, 37) • Shake head "no" when offered more pasta. (18 mos.; Meisels and others 2003, 37) • Make a big pile of trucks and a little pile of trucks. • Use hand motions or words to indicate "All gone" when finished eating. (12–19 mos.; Parks 2004, 122) • Put three cars in a row.	• Pick out one object from a box or point to the picture with only one of something. (Scaled score of 10 for 35:16–36:15 mos.; Bayley 2006, 97; 24–30 mos.; Parks 2004) • Reach into bowl and take out two pieces of pear when the infant care teacher says, "Just take two." (30–36 mos.; Parks 2004) • Start counting with one, sometimes pointing to the same item twice when counting, or using numbers out of order; for example, "one, two, three, five, eight." (36 mos.; *Engaging Young Children* 2004, 178) • Use fingers to count a small number of items. (around 36 mos.; Coplan 1993, 3) • Look at a plate and quickly respond "two," without having to count, when the infant care teacher asks how many pieces of cheese there are. (36 mos.; *Engaging Young Children* 2004, 178) • Hold up two fingers when asked, "Show me two" or "How old are you?" (36 mos.; *Engaging Young Children* 2004, 178; by 36 mos.; American Academy of Pediatrics 2004, 308) • Identify "more" with collections of up to four items, without needing to count them. (36 mos.; *Engaging Young Children* 2004, 31 and 180) • Use more specific words to communicate how many, such as a little or a lot. (Hulit and Howard 2006, 186)

Chart continues on next page.

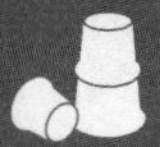

Number Sense

Behaviors leading up to the foundation (4 to 7 months)	Behaviors leading up to the foundation (9 to 17 months)	Behaviors leading up to the foundation (19 to 35 months)
During this period, the child may: • Explore toys with hands and mouth. (3–6 mos.; Parks 2004, 10) • Reach for second toy but may not grasp it when already hold-ing one toy in the other hand. (5–6.5 mos.; Parks 2004, 49; scaled score of 10 for 5:16–6:15 mos.; Bayley 2006, 55) • Transfer a toy from one hand to the other. (5.5–7 mos.; Parks 2004) • Reach for, grasp, and hold onto a toy with one hand when already holding a different toy in the other hand. (Scaled score of 10 for 6:16–7:15 mos.; Bayley 2006, 56) • Track visually the path of a moving object. (6–8 mos.; Parks 2004, 64)	During this period, the child may: • Try to hold onto two toys with one hand while reaching for a third desired toy, even if not successful. (Scaled score of 9 for 10:16–11:15 mos.; Bayley 2006, 58; 8–10 mos.; Parks 2004, 50) • Hold a block in each hand and bang them together. (8.5–12 mos.; Parks 2004) • Put several pegs into a plastic container and then dump them into a pile. (12–13 mos.; Parks 2004, 65)	During this period, the child may: • Get two cups from the cupboard when playing in the housekeep-ing area with a friend. (21 mos.; Mix, Huttenlocher, and Levine 2002) • Look at or point to the child with one piece of apple left on his napkin when the infant care teacher asks, "Who has just one piece of apple?" (24–30 mos.; Parks 2004, 74) • Give the infant care teacher one cracker from a pile of many when she asks for "one." (25–30 mos.; Parks 2004; scaled score of 10 for 28:16–30:15 mos.; Bayley 2006, 73)

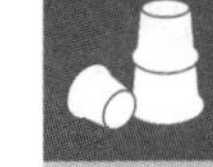

Foundation: Classification

The developing ability to group, sort, categorize, connect, and have expectations of objects and people according to their attributes

8 months	*18 months*	*36 months*
At around eight months of age, children distinguish between familiar and unfamiliar people, places, and objects, and explore the differences between them. (Barrera and Mauer 1981)	At around 18 months of age, children show awareness when objects are in some way connected to each other, match two objects that are the same, and separate a pile of objects into two groups based on one attribute. (Mandler and McDonough 1998)	At around 36 months of age, children group objects into multiple piles based on one attribute at a time, put things that are similar but not identical into one group, and may label each grouping, even though sometimes these labels are overgeneralized. (36 mos.; Mandler and McDonough 1993)
For example, the child may:	**For example, the child may:**	**For example, the child may:**
• Explore how one toy feels and then explore how another toy feels. • Stare at an unfamiliar person and move toward a familiar person.	• Look at the crayons before choosing a color. (12–18 mos.; Parks 2004, 77) • Choose usually to play with the blue ball even though there is a red one just like it. (12–18 mos.; Parks 2004, 77) • Pick the toy car from the bin filled with toy dishes. (15–18 mos.; Parks 2004; 77) • Pack the baby doll's blanket, brush, bottle, and clothes into a backpack. (15–19 mos.; Parks 2004, 77) • Match two identical toys; for example, find another fire truck when the infant care teacher asks, "Can you find a truck just like that one?" (15–19 mos.; Parks 2004; 77) • Place all toy cars on one side of the rug and all blocks on the other side. (15–18 mos.; Parks 2004, 77)	• Identify a few colors when they are named; for example, get a red ball from the bin of multicolored balls when the infant care teacher asks for the red one. (Scaled score of 10 for 34:16–36:15 mos.; Bayley 2006, 97; 33 mos.+; Parks 2004, 79) • Make three piles of tangrams in various shapes, such as a circle, square, and triangle. (30–36 mos.; Parks 2004, 79) • Pick two big bears from a bowl containing two big bears and two small bears, even if the big bears are different colors. (Scaled score of 10 for 30:16–33:15 mos.; Bayley 2006, 74) • Sort primary-colored blocks into three piles: a red pile, a yellow pile, and a blue one. (33 mos.+; Parks 2004, 79; 32 mos.; Bayley 2006) • Point to different pictures of houses in a book even though all of the houses look different. (30–36 mos.; Parks 2004, 79) • Put all the soft stuffed animals in one pile and all the hard plastic toy animals in another pile and label the piles "soft animals" and "hard animals." (18–36 mos.; Lally and others 1995, 78–79) • Call all four-legged animals at the farm "cows," even though some are actually sheep and others horses. (18–36 mos.; Lally and others 1995, 78–79)

Chart continues on next page.

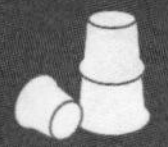

Classification

Behaviors leading up to the foundation (4 to 7 months)	Behaviors leading up to the foundation (9 to 17 months)	Behaviors leading up to the foundation (19 to 35 months)
During this period, the child may: • Explore toys with hands and mouth. (3–6 mos.; Parks 2004, 10) • Bang a toy on the table. (5.5–7 mos.; Parks 2004, 25) • Touch different objects (e.g., hard or soft) differently.	During this period, the child may: • Roll a car back and forth on the floor, then roll a ball. (6–11 mos.; Parks 2004, 26) • Use two items that go together; for example, brush a doll's hair with a brush, put a spoon in a bowl, or use a hammer to pound an object. (9–15 mos.; Parks 2004, 26–27; by 12 mos.; American Academy of Pediatrics 2004, 243) • Put the red blocks together when the infant care teacher asks, "Which blocks go together?"	During this period, the child may: • Point to or indicate the realistic-looking plastic cow when the infant care teacher holds up a few toy animals and says, "Who says, 'moo'?" (18–22 mos.; Parks 2004; 85) • Sort three different kinds of toys; for example, put the puzzle pieces in the puzzle box, the blocks in the block bin, and the toy animals in the basket during clean-up time. (19–24 mos.; Parks 2004, 77) • Show understanding of what familiar objects are supposed to be used for, such as knowing that a hat is for wearing or a tricycle is for riding. (Scaled score of 10 for 23:16–25:15 mos.; Bayley 2006, 93) • Pick a matching card from a pile of cards. (Scaled score of 10 for 24:16–25:15 mos.; Bayley 2006, 70) • Point to or indicate all the green cups at the lunch table. (26 mos.; Bayley 2006) • Call the big animals "mama" and the small animals "baby." (27 mos.; Bayley 2006) • Help the infant care teacher sort laundry into two piles: whites and colors. (28 mos.; Hart and Risley 1999, 95) • Put the red marker back in the red can, the blue marker back in the blue can, and the yellow marker back in the yellow can when finished coloring. (Scaled score of 10 for 26:16–28:15 mos.; Bayley 2006, 71) • Match one shape to another shape. (26–29 mos.; Parks 2004, 78; 26–30 mos.; Parks 2004)

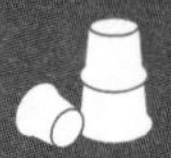

Foundation: Symbolic Play

The developing ability to use actions, objects, or ideas to represent other actions, objects, or ideas

8 months	*18 months*	*36 months*
At around 8 months of age, children become familiar with objects and actions through active exploration. Children also build knowledge of people, action, objects, and ideas through observation. (Fenson and others 1976; Rogoff and others 2003)	At around 18 months of age, children use one object to represent another object and engage in one or two simple actions of pretend play.	At around 36 months of age, children engage in make-believe play involving several sequenced steps, assigned roles, and an overall plan and sometimes pretend by imagining an object without needing the concrete object present. (30–36 mos.; Parks 2004, 29)
For example, the child may:	**For example, the child may:**	**For example, the child may:**
• Cause toys to make noise by shaking, banging, and squeezing them. (5.5–8 mos.; Parks 2004, 58; by 12 mos.; American Academy of Pediatrics 2004, 243) • Roll car back and forth on floor. (6–11 mos.; Parks 2004, 26)	• Pretend to drink from an empty cup by making slurping noises and saying "ah" when finished. (Segal 2004, 39) • Begin to engage in pretend play by using a play spoon to stir in the kitchen area. (12–18 mos.; Lerner and Ciervo 2003) • Pretend that the banana is a telephone by picking it up, holding it to the ear, and saying, "Hi!" (12–18 mos.; Lerner and Ciervo 2003) • Laugh at an older brother when he puts a bowl on his head like a hat. (12–18 mos.; Parks 2004, 317) • Imitate a few steps of adult behavior during play; for example, pretend to feed the baby doll with the toy spoon and bowl. (15–18 mos.; Parks 2004, 27) • Use a rectangular wooden block as a phone. (18–24 mos.; Parks 2004, 28)	• Assign roles to self and others when playing in the dramatic play area (for example, "I'll be the daddy, you be the baby"), even though the child may not stay in her role throughout the play sequence. (30–36 mos.; Parks 2004, 29; 24 mos.; Segal 2004, 43) • Line up a row of chairs and communicate, "All aboard! The train is leaving." (36 mos.; Vygotsky 1978, 111) • Use two markers to represent people in the dollhouse by moving them around as if they were walking. (36 mos.; Vygotsky 1978, 111) • Stir "cake batter" while holding an imaginary spoon or serve an invisible burrito on a plate. (30–36 mos.; Parks 2004, 29; scaled score of 10 for 27:16–29:15 mos.; Bayley 2006, 69) • Communicate with self during pretend play to describe actions to self; for example, "Now I stir the soup." (Hart and Risley 1999, 125) • Plan with other children what they are going to pretend before starting to play; for example, "Let's play doggies!" (Segal 2004, 39; 36 mos.; Meisels and others 2003, 74) • Pretend to be a baby during dramatic play because there is a new baby at home. (36 mos.; Meisels and others 2003, 73) • Build a small town with blocks and then use the toy fire truck to pretend to put out a fire in the town. (By 36 mos.; American Academy of Pediatrics 2004, 309)

Chart continues on next page.

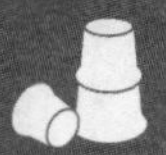

Symbolic Play

Behaviors leading up to the foundation (4 to 7 months)	Behaviors leading up to the foundation (9 to 17 months)	Behaviors leading up to the foundation (19 to 35 months)
During this period, the child may: • Explore toys with hands and mouth. (3–6 mos.; Parks 2004, 10)	During this period, the child may: • Use two items that go together; for example, brush a doll's hair with brush, put a spoon in a bowl, or use a hammer to pound an object through a hole. (9–15 mos.; Parks 2004, 26–27) • Use objects in pretend play the way they were intended to be used; for example, pretend to drink coffee or tea from play coffee cup. (Scaled score of 10 for 15:16–16:15 mos.; Bayley 2006, 62)	During this period, the child may: • Use the stuffed animals to play "veterinarian" one day and then to play "farmer" the next day. (18–24 mos.; Lerner and Ciervo 2003) • Communicate "Time for night-night" to a doll while playing house. (22–24 mos.; Parks 2004, 133) • Complete three or more actions in a sequence of pretend play so the actions have a beginning, middle, and end, such as giving the baby doll a bath, putting his pajamas on, and putting him to sleep. (24–30 mos.; Parks 2004, 28; by 36 mos.; American Academy of Pediatrics 2004, 309; scaled score of 10 for 29:16–30:15 mos.; Bayley 2006, 73) • Pretend that the doll or stuffed animal has feelings, such as making a whining noise to indicate that the stuffed puppy is sad. (24–30 mos.; Parks 2004, 28) • Make the stuffed animals move, as if they were alive, during pretend play. (24–30 mos.; Parks 2004, 28) • Engage in extended pretend play that has a theme, such as birthday party or doctor. (24–30 mos.; Parks 2004, 29) • Use abstract things to represent other things in pretend play; for example, use dough or sand to represent a birthday cake and sticks or straws to represent candles. (24–30 mos.; Parks 2004, 29; scaled score of 10 for 24:16–25:15 mos.; Bayley 2006, 70; Segal 2004, 39)

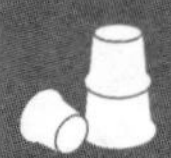

Foundation: Attention Maintenance

The developing ability to attend to people and things while interacting with others and exploring the environment and play materials

8 months	*18 months*	*36 months*
At around eight months of age, children pay attention to different things and people in the environment in specific, distinct ways. (Bronson 2000, 64)	At around 18 months of age, children rely on order and predictability in the environment to help organize their thoughts and focus attention. (Bronson 2000, 191)	At around 36 months of age, children sometimes demonstrate the ability to pay attention to more than one thing at a time.
For example, the child may:	**For example, the child may:**	**For example, the child may:**
• Play with one toy for a few minutes before focusing on a different toy. (6–9 mos.; Parks 2004, 12 and 26; 8 mos.; American Academy of Pediatrics 2004, 241) • Focus on a desired toy that is just out of reach while repeatedly reaching for it. (5–9 mos.; Parks 2004, 49) • Show momentary attention to board books with bright colors and simple shapes. • Attend to the play of other children. • Put toy animals into a clear container, dump them out, and then fill the container up again. (8 mos.; Meisels and others 2003, 21) • Stop moving, to focus on the infant care teacher when she starts to interact with the child.	• Expect favorite songs to be sung the same way each time and protest if the infant care teacher changes the words. • Insist on following the same bedtime routine every night. • Nod and take the infant care teacher's hand when the teacher says, "I know you are sad because Shanti is using the book right now, and you would like a turn. Shall we go to the book basket and find another one to read together?"	• Realize, during clean-up time, that he has put a car in the block bin and return to put it in the proper place. • Search for and find a favorite book and ask the infant care teacher to read it. • Pound the play dough with a hammer while talking with a peer.
Behaviors leading up to the foundation (4 to 7 months)	**Behaviors leading up to the foundation (9 to 17 months)**	**Behaviors leading up to the foundation (19 to 35 months)**
During this period, the child may: • Remain calm and focused on people, interesting toys, or interesting sounds for a minute or so. (1–6 mos.; Parks 2004, 9) • Explore a toy by banging, mouthing, or looking at it. (Scaled score of 9 for 3:26–4:05 mos.; Bayley 2006, 52)	During this period, the child may: • Pay attention to the infant care teacher's voice without being distracted by other noises in the room. (9–11 mos.; Parks 2004; 12) • Focus on one toy or activity for a while when really interested. (By 12 mos.; American Academy of Pediatrics 2004, 241)	During this period, the child may: • Play alone with toys for several minutes at a time before moving on to different activity. (18–24 mos.; Parks 2004, 15) • Sit in a parent's lap to read a book together. (Scaled score of 10 for 21:16–22:15 mos.; Bayley 2006)

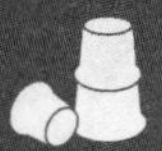

Foundation: Understanding of Personal Care Routines

The developing ability to understand and participate in personal care routines

8 months	*18 months*	*36 months*
At around eight months of age, children are responsive during the steps of personal care routines. (CDE 2005)	At around 18 months of age, children show awareness of familiar personal care routines and participate in the steps of these routines. (CDE 2005)	At around 36 months of age, children initiate and follow through with some personal care routines. (CDE 2005)
For example, the child may:	**For example, the child may:**	**For example, the child may:**
• Turn head away as the infant care teacher reaches with a tissue to wipe the child's nose. (8 mos.; Meisels and others 2003, 20) • Kick legs in anticipation of a diaper change and then quiet down as the parent wipes the child's bottom. (CDE 2005) • Pay attention to her hands as the infant care teacher holds them under running water and helps rub them together with soap. (CDE 2005)	• Go to the sink when the infant care teacher says that it is time to wash hands. (Scaled score of 10 for 17:16–18:15 mos.; Bayley 2006, 90; 12–18 mos.; Lerner and Ciervo 2003; 12 mos.; Coplan 1993, 2; by 24 mos.; American Academy of Pediatrics 2004; 24 mos.; Meisels and others 2003, 46) • Get a tissue when the infant care teacher says, "Please go get a tissue. We need to wipe your nose." (18 mos.; Meisels and others 2003, 36) • Move toward the door to the playground after seeing the infant care teacher put his coat on. (18 mos.; Meisels and others 2003, 38) • Put snack dishes in the sink and the bib in the hamper after eating. • Have trouble settling down for a nap until the infant care teacher reads a story, because that is the naptime routine. (12–18 mos.; Parks 2004, 317)	• Go to the sink and wash hands after seeing snacks being set out on the table. (CDE 2005) • Get a tissue to wipe own nose or bring the tissue to the infant care teacher for help when the child feels that his nose needs to be wiped. (CDE 2005) • Take a wet shirt off when needing to put on a dry one. (36 mos.; Meisels and others 2003, 76) • Help set the table for lunchtime. (36 mos.; Meisels and others 2003, 77)
Behaviors leading up to the foundation (4 to 7 months)	**Behaviors leading up to the foundation (9 to 17 months)**	**Behaviors leading up to the foundation (19 to 35 months)**
During this period, the child may: • Anticipate being fed upon seeing the infant care teacher approach with a bottle. • Hold onto the bottle while being fed by the infant care teacher. (4 mos.; Meisels and others 2003, 14)	During this period, the child may: • Cooperate during a diaper change by lifting her bottom. (10.5–12 mos.; Parks 2004) • Grab the spoon as the infant care teacher tries to feed the child. (12 mos.; Meisels and others 2003, 31) • Raise arms when the infant care teacher tries to put a dry shirt on the child. (12 mos.; Meisels and others 2003)	During this period, the child may: • Drink from a cup without spilling much. (24 mos.; Meisels and others 2003, 52) • Try to put on own socks. (24 mos.; Meisels and others 2003, 52) • Pull her shoes off at naptime. (24 mos.; Meisels and others 2003, 52)

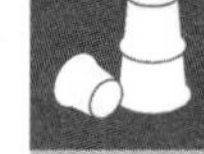

References

American Academy of Pediatrics. 2004. *Caring for Your Baby and Young Child: Birth to Age 5* (Fourth edition). Edited by S. P. Shelov and R. E. Hannemann. New York: Bantam Books.

Apfel, N. H., and S. Provence. 2001. *Manual for the Infant-Toddler and Family Instrument (ITFI).* Baltimore, MD: Paul H. Brookes Publishing.

Baillargeon, R. 2004. "Infants' Physical World," *Current Directions in Psychological Science,* Vol. 13, No. 3, 89–94.

Bard, K., and C. Russell. 1999. "Evolutionary Foundations of Imitation: Social-Cognitive and Developmental Aspects of Imitative Processes in Non-Human Primates," in *Imitation in Infancy: Cambridge Studies in Cognitive and Perceptual Development.* Edited by J. Nadel and G. Butterworth. Cambridge, UK: Cambridge University Press.

Barrera, M. E., and Mauer, D. 1981. "The Perception of Facial Expressions by the Three-month-old." *Child Development,* Vol. 52, 203–6.

Bauer, P. 2002a. "Early Memory Development," in *Handbook of Cognitive Development.* Edited by U. Goswami. Oxford, England: Blackwell.

Bauer, P. 2002b. "Long-Term Recall Memory: Behavioral and Neuro-Developmental Changes in the First Two Years of Life," *Current Directions in Psychological Science,* Vol. 11, No. 4, 137–41.

Bauer, P. 2004. "Getting Explicit Memory off the Ground: Steps Toward Construction of a Neuro-Developmental Account of Changes in the First Two Years of Life," *Developmental Review,* Vol. 24, 347–73.

Bauer, P. 2007. "Recall in Infancy: A Neurodevelopmental Account," *Current Directions in Psychological Science,* Vol. 16, No. 3, 142–46.

Bauer, P. J., and J. M. Mandler. 1989. "One Thing Follows Another: Effects of Temporal Structure on 1- to 2-Year Olds' Recall of Events," *Developmental Psychology,* Vol. 8, 241–63.

Bayley, N. 2006. *Bayley Scales of Infant and Toddler Development* (Third edition). San Antonio, TX: Harcourt Assessment, Inc.

Brazelton, T. B. 1992. *Touchpoints: Your Child's Emotional and Behavioral Development.* New York: Perseus Books.

Bronson, M. 2000. *Self-regulation in Early Childhood: Nature and Nurture.* New York: Guilford Press.

Brooks-Gunn, J., and G. Duncan. 1997. "The Effects of Poverty on Children," *The Future of Children,* Vol. 7, No. 2, 55–71.

Butterworth, G. 1999. "Neonatal Imitation: Existence, Mechanisms and Motives," *Imitation in Infancy: Cambridge Studies in Cognitive and Perceptual Development.* Edited by J. Nadel and C. Butterworth. New York: Cambridge University Press.

California Department of Education (CDE). 2005. "Desired Results Developmental Profile (DRDP)," Sacramento, CA: California Department of Education. http://www.cde.ca.gov/sp/cd/ci/desiredresults.asp (accessed February 7, 2007).

Carey, S. 2001. "On the Very Possibility of Discontinuities in Conceptual Development," in *Language, Brain, and Cognitive Development: Essays in Honor of Jacques Mehler.* Edited by E. Dupoux. Cambridge, MA: MIT Press.

Clements, D. H. 2004. "Major Themes and Recommendations," in *Engaging Young Children in Mathematics: Standards for Early Childhood Educators.* Edited by D. H. Clements and J. Samara. Mahwah, NJ: Lawrence Erlbaum Associates.

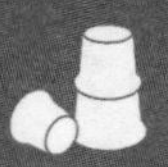

Coplan, J. 1993. *Early Language Milestone Scale: Examiner's Manual* (Second edition). Austin, TX: Pro-ed.

Engaging Young Children in Mathematics: Standards for Early Childhood Mathematics Education. 2004. Edited by D. H. Clements and J. Sarama. Mahwah, NJ: Lawrence Erlbaum Associates.

Fenson, L., and others. 1976. "The Developmental Progression of Manipulative Play in the First Two Years," *Child Development,* Vol. 47, No. 1, 232–36.

Fogel, A. 2001. *Infancy: Infant, Family, and Society* (Fourth edition). Belmont, CA: Wadsworth/Thomson Learning.

Fuson, K. C. 1988. *Children's Counting and Concepts of Number.* New York: Springer-Verlag.

Gallistel, C. R., and R. Gelman. 1992. "Preverbal and Verbal Counting and Computation," *Cognition,* Vol. 44, No. 1–2, 43–74.

Gelman, R., and C. R. Gallistel. 1978. *The Child's Understanding of Number.* Oxford, England: Harvard University Press.

Ginsburg, H. P., and S. Opper. 1988. *Piaget's Theory of Intellectual Development* (Third edition). Englewood Cliffs, NJ: Prentice Hall.

Gopnik, A.; A. Meltzoff; and P. K. Kuhl. 1999. *The Scientist in the Crib: Minds, Brains, and How Children Learn.* New York: William Morrow.

Gowen, J. W. March, 1995. "Research in Review: The Early Development of Symbolic Play," *Young Children,* Vol. 50, No. 3, 75–84.

Hart, B., and T. R. Risley. 1999. *The Social World of Children: Learning to Talk.* Baltimore, MD: Paul H. Brookes Publishing.

Howe, M., and M. Courage. 1993. "On Resolving the Enigma of Infantile Amnesia," *Psychological Bulletin,* Vol. 113, No. 2, 305–26.

Hulit, L. M., and M. R. Howard. 2006. *Born to Talk: An Introduction to Speech and Language Development* (Fourth edition). New York: Pearson Education.

Kail, R. 1990. *The Development of Memory in Children* (Third edition). New York: W. H. Freeman.

Lally, J. R., and others. 1995. *Caring for Infants and Toddlers in Groups: Developmentally Appropriate Practice.* Washington, DC: Zero to Three Press.

Legerstee, M. 1997. "Contingency Effects of People and Objects on Subsequent Cognitive Functioning in Three-Month-Old Infants," *Social Development,* Vol. 6, No. 3, 307–21.

Lerner, C., and A. L. Dombro. 2000. *Learning and Growing Together: Understanding and Supporting Your Child's Development.* Washington, DC: Zero to Three Press.

Lerner, C., and L. A. Ciervo. 2003. *Healthy Minds: Nurturing Children's Development from 0 to 36 Months.* Washington, DC: Zero to Three Press and American Academy of Pediatrics.

Madole, K., and L. Oakes. 1999. "Making Sense of Infant Categorization: Stable Processes and Changing Representations," *Developmental Review,* Vol. 19, No. 2, 263–96.

Mandler, J. M. 2000. "Perceptual and Conceptual Processes in Infancy," *Journal of Cognition and Development,* Vol. 1, No. 1, 3–36.

Mandler, J., and L. McDonough. 1993. "Concept Formation in Infancy," *Cognitive Development,* Vol. 8, No. 3, 291–318.

Mandler, J., and L. McDonough. 1998. "On Developing a Knowledge Base in Infancy," *Developmental Psychology,* Vol. 34, No. 6, 1274–88.

Mangione, P. L.; J. R. Lally; and S. Signer. 1992. *Discoveries of Infancy: Cognitive Development and Learning.* Sacramento, CA: Far West Laboratory and California Department of Education.

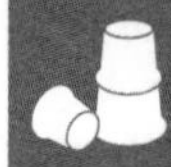

Mareschal, D., and R. French. 2000. "Mechanisms of Categorization in Infancy," *Infancy*, Vol. 1, No. 1, 59–76.

Meltzoff, A. N., and M. K. Moore. 1983. "Newborn Infants Imitate Adult Facial Gestures," *Child Development*, Vol. 54, 702–9.

Meltzoff, A. N., and M. K. Moore. 1989. "Imitation in Newborn Infants: Exploring the Range of Gestures Imitated and the Underlying Mechanisms," *Developmental Psychology*, Vol. 25, No. 6, 954–62.

Meltzoff, A. N., and M. K. Moore. 1999. "Persons and Representation: Why Infant Imitation Is Important for Theories of Human Development, " in *Imitation in Infancy: Cambridge Studies in Cognitive and Perceptual Development.* Edited by J. Nadel and G. Butterworth. New York: Cambridge University Press.

Meisels, S. J., and others. 2003. *The Ounce Scale: Standards for the Developmental Profiles (Birth–42 Months).* New York: Pearson Early Learning.

Mix, K.; J. Huttenlocher; and S. Levine. 2002. *Quantitative Development in Infancy and Early Childhood.* New York: Oxford University Press.

Moser, R. F. 1995. "Caregivers' Corner. Fantasy Play in the Sandbox," *Young Children*, Vol. 51, No. 1, 83–84.

National Research Council and Institute of Medicine. 2000. *From Neurons to Neighborhoods: The Science of Early Childhood Development.* Committee on Integrating the Science of Early Childhood Development. Edited by J. Shonkoff and D. Phillips. Washington, DC: National Academies Press.

O'Brien, M. 1997. *Meeting Individual and Special Needs: Inclusive Child Care for Infants and Toddlers.* Baltimore, MD: Paul H. Brookes Publishing.

Parks, S. 2004. *Inside HELP: Hawaii Early Learning Profile: Administration and Reference Manual.* Palo Alto, CA: VORT Corporation.

Perry, J. P. May, 2003. "Making Sense of Outdoor Pretend Play," *Young Children*, Vol. 58, No. 3, 26–30.

Rogoff, B. 1990. *Apprenticeship in Thinking: Cognitive Development in Social Context.* New York: Oxford University Press.

Rogoff, B., and P. Chavajay. 1995. "What's Become of Research on the Cultural Basis of Cognitive Development?" *American Psychologist*, Vol. 50, No. 10, 859–77.

Rogoff, B., and others. 2003. "Firsthand Learning Through Intent Participation," *Annual Review of Psychology*, Vol. 54, 175–203.

Ruff, H., and M. Rothbart. 1996. *Attention in Early Development: Themes and Variations.* New York: Oxford University Press.

Segal, M. 2004. "The Roots and Fruits of Pretending," in *Children's Play: The Roots of Reading.* Edited by E. F. Zigler, D. G. Singer, and S. J. Bishop-Josef. Washington, DC: Zero to Three Press.

Siegel, D.J. 1999. *The Developing Mind: How Relationships and the Brain Interact to Shape Who We Are.* New York: Guilford Press.

Starkey, P., and R. G. Cooper. 1980. "Perception of Numbers by Human Infants," *Science*, Vol. 210, No. 4473, 1033–35.

Starkey, P.; E. S. Spelke; and R. Gelman. 1990. "Numerical Abstraction by Human Infants," *Cognition*, Vol. 36, No. 2, 97–128.

Sternberg, R. J., and E. L. Grigorenko. 2004. "Why We Need to Explore Development in Its Cultural Context," *Merrill-Palmer Quarterly*, Vol. 50, No. 3, 369–86.

Vygotsky, L. S. 1978. *Mind in Society: The Development of Higher Psychological Processes.* Cambridge, MA: Harvard University Press.

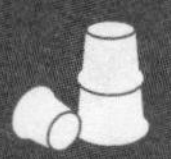

Whitehurst, G., and C. Lonigan. 1998. "Child Development and Emergent Literacy," *Child Development*, Vol. 69, No. 3, 848–72.

Wynn, K. 1998. "Numerical Competence in Infants," in *The Development of Mathematical Skills.* Edited by C. Donlad. Hove, East Sussex, UK: Psychology Press.

Youngblade, L. M., and J. Dunn. 1995. "Individual Differences in Young Children's Pretend Play with Mother and Sibling: Links to Relationships and Understanding of Other People's Feelings and Beliefs," *Child Development*, Vol. 66, 1472–92.

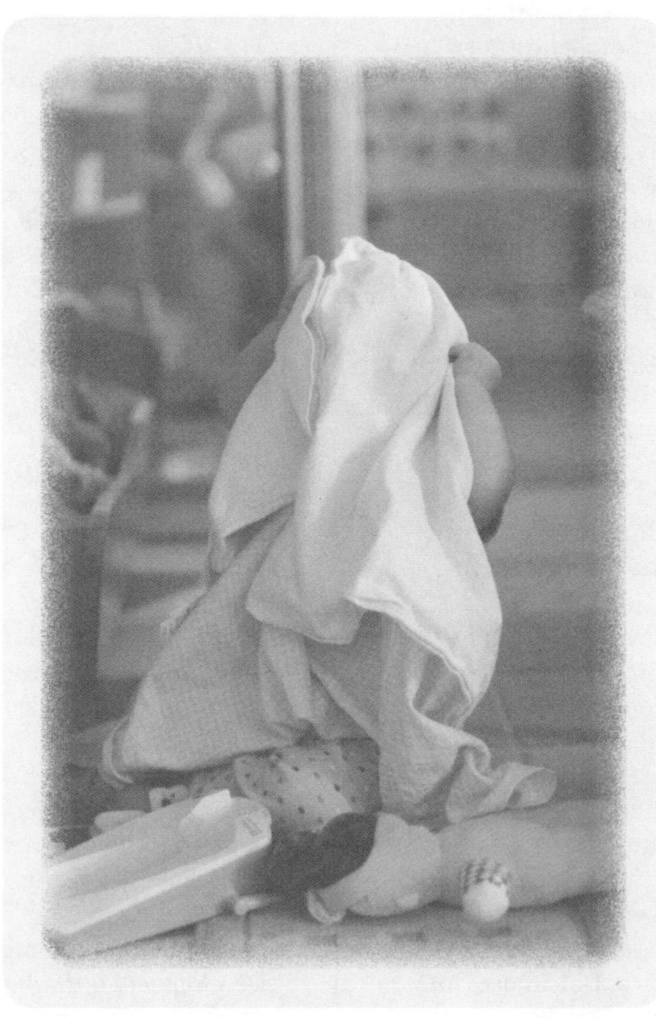

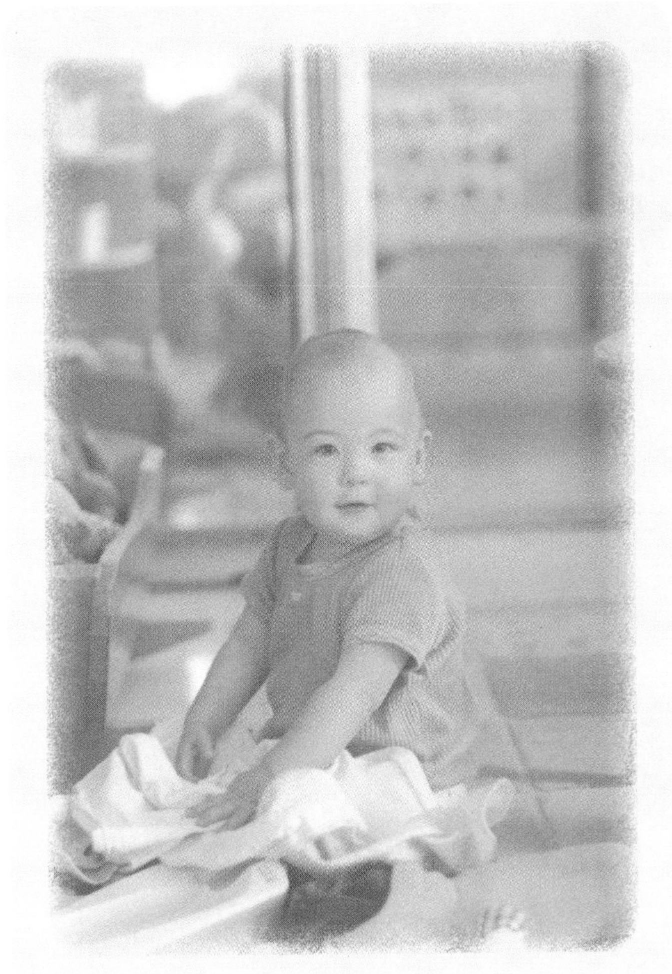

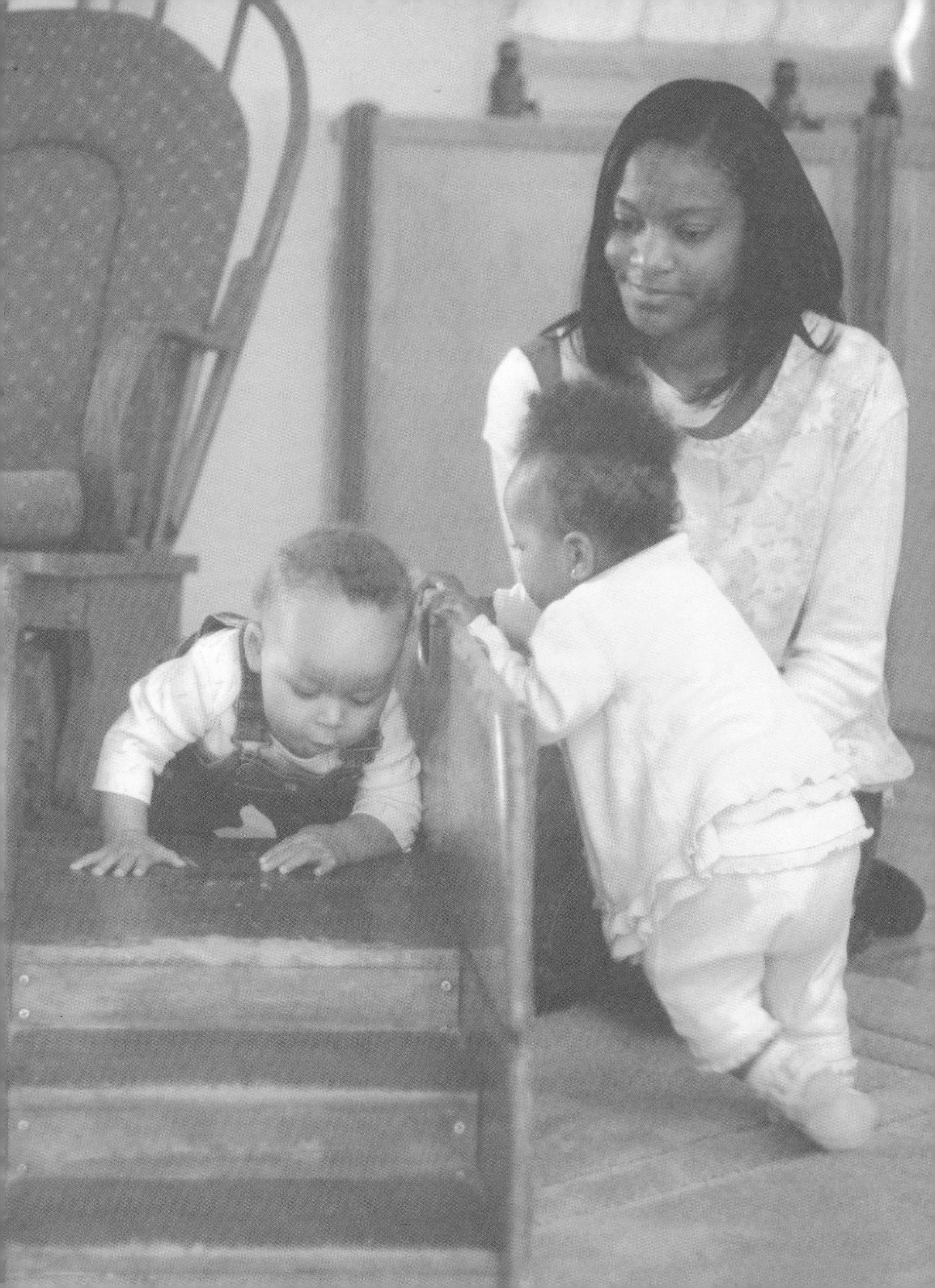

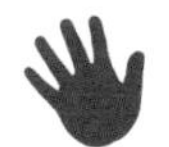

Perceptual and Motor Development

Perception refers to the process of taking in, organizing, and interpreting sensory information. Perception is multimodal, with multiple sensory inputs contributing to motor responses (Bertenthal 1996). An infant's turning his head in response to the visual and auditory cues of the sight of a face and the sound of a voice exemplifies this type of perception. Intersensory redundancy, "the fact that the senses provide overlapping information . . . is a cornerstone of perceptual development" (Bahrick, Lickliter, and Flom 2004).

"Motor development refers to changes in children's ability to control their body's movements, from infants' first spontaneous waving and kicking movements to the adaptive control of reaching, locomotion, and complex sport skills" (Adolph, Weise, and Marin 2003, 134). The term *motor behavior* describes all movements of the body, including movements of the eyes (as in the gaze), and the infant's developing control of the head. Gross motor actions include the movement of large limbs or the whole body, as in walking. Fine motor behaviors include the use of fingers to grasp and manipulate objects. Motor behaviors such as reaching, touching, and grasping are forms of exploratory activity (Adolph 1997).

As infants develop increasing motor competence, they use perceptual information to inform their choices about which motor actions to take (Adolph and Joh 2007). For example, they may adjust their crawling or walking in response to the rigidity, slipperiness, or slant of surfaces (Adolph 1997). Motor movements, including movements of the eyes, arms, legs, and hands, provide most of the perceptual information infants receive (Adolph and Berger 2006). Young children's bodies undergo remarkable changes in the early childhood years. In describing this development, Adolph and Avolio (2000, 1148) state, "Newborns are extremely top-heavy with large heads and torsos and short, weak legs. As infants grow, their body fat and muscle mass are redistributed. In contrast to newborns, toddlers' bodies have a more cylindrical shape, and they have a larger ratio of muscle mass to body fat, especially in the legs." These changes in weight, size, percentage of body fat, and muscle strength provide perceptual/motor challenges to infants as they practice a variety of actions (Adolph and Berger 2006). This dramatic physical development occurs within the broad context of overall development. As infants master each challenge, their perceptual and motor behavior reflects their ever-present interpersonal orientation and social environment.

The extent and variety of infant perceptual and motor behavior are remarkable. Infants and toddlers spend a significant part of their days engaged in motor behavior of one type or another. By three and a half months of age, infants have made between three and six million eye movements during their waking hours (Haith, Hazen, and Goodman 1988). Infants who crawl and walk have been found to spend roughly half of their waking hours involved in motor behavior, approximately five to six hours per day (Adolph and Joh 2007, 11). On a daily basis infants who are walking ". . . take more than 9,000 steps and travel the distance of more than 29 football fields. They travel over nearly a dozen different indoor and outdoor surfaces varying in friction, rigidity and texture. They visit nearly every room in their homes and they engage in balance and locomotion in the context of varied activities" (Adolph and Berger 2006, 181).

Early research in motor development involved detailed observational studies that documented the progression of infant motor skills and presented an understanding of infant motor behavior as a sequence of universal, biologically programmed steps (Adolph and Berger 2006; Bertenthal and Boker 1997; Bushnell and Boudreau 1993; Pick 1989). In comparison, current research in motor development often emphasizes action in the context of behavior and development in the perceptual, cognitive, and social domains (Pick 1989). In particular, contemporary accounts of infant motor development address (1) the strong relationship between perception and action (Bertenthal 1996; Gibson 1988; Thelen 1995), (2) the relationship between actions and the environment (Gibson 1988; Thelen 1995), and (3) the importance of motives in motor behavior, notably social and explorative motives (von Hofsten 2007). Although historical approaches may encourage professionals to focus on the relationship between growing perceptual/motor skills and the child's increasingly sophisticated manipulation and understanding of objects, contemporary understanding suggests the value of observation of this progression. How these developing behaviors and abilities play a role in the social/emotional aspects of the child's life and functioning, such as forming early relationships and building an understanding of others, may be noteworthy.

The contemporary view suggests that thinking about perceptual/motor development can be inclusive of infants and toddlers with disabilities or other special needs. Children whose disabilities affect their perceptual or motor development still want to explore and interact with the people and environment around them. Although the perceptual and motor development of children with disabilities or other special needs may follow a pathway that differs from typical developmental trajectories, sensitive and responsive caregivers can provide alternative ways in which to engage children's drive to explore, building on their interests and strengths and supporting their overall physical and psychological health.

Pioneering researchers in infant motor development used novel and painstaking methods to study the progression of infant skill acquisition (Adolph and Berger 2005; Adolph 2008). Their findings were presented for both professionals and the public in the form of milestone charts that depicted motor skill acquisition as a clear progression through a series of predictable stages related to chronological age (Adolph 2008; Adolph, Weise, and Marin 2003). More recent research in the area of perceptual and motor development has indicated substantial variability between children in the pathways to acquiring major motor milestones such as sitting and walking (Adolph 1997; Adolph 2008). Each child may take a unique developmental pathway toward attainment of major motor milestones (Adolph and Joh 2007). Crawling, for example, is not a universal stage. Research clearly shows that not all children crawl before they walk (Adolph 2008). Although most children walk independently around age one, the normal range for acquisition of this behavior in western cultures is very broad, between 9 and 17 months of age (Adolph 2008). Age has traditionally been treated as the primary predictor of when landmark motor behaviors occur, but studies now indicate that experience may be a stronger predictor than age is in the emergence of both crawling (Adolph and Joh 2007) and walking (Adolph, Vereijken, and Shrout 2003).

It is important to recognize that, though developmental charts may show motor development unfolding in the form of a smooth upward progression toward mastery, the development of individual children often does not follow a smooth upward trajectory. In fact, "detours" and steps backward are common as development unfolds (Adolph and Berger 2006, 173). Infant motor development can be understood as a process in which change occurs as the infant actively adapts to varying circumstances and new tasks (Thelen 1995). Thelen (1994) demonstrated this experimentally in her well-known study in which three-month-old babies, still too young to coordinate their movements to be able to sit, reach, or crawl, learned to coordinate their kicks in order to engage in the novel task of making a mobile move. Cultural and historical factors, including caregivers' behavior, also affect the ways in which infants engage in motor behaviors. For example, Adolph and Berger (2005) observed that mothers in Jamaica and Mali "train" infants to sit by propping up three- to four-month-old infants with pillows in a special hole in the ground designed to provide back support.

For years, researchers, educators, and early childhood professionals have emphasized the interrelatedness of the developmental domains. The current research supports an even greater appreciation of the profound role of interrelatedness and interdependence of factors, domains, and processes in development (Diamond 2007). The developmental domains are linked not only with one another, but also with factors such as culture, social relationships, experience, physical health,

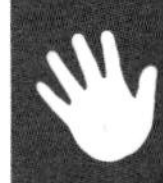

mental health, and brain functioning (Diamond 2007). In the case of perceptual and motor behavior, Diamond (2007) has observed that perception, motor behavior, and cognition occur in the context of culture, emotion, social relationships, and experience, which in turn influence physical and mental health as well as overall brain functioning. Bertenthal (1996) has proposed that perception and motor action are interrelated rather than autonomous processes. They may be best viewed as different components of an action system. Common behaviors such as reaching and turning the head for visual tracking illustrate the interrelatedness of the motor, perceptual, cognitive, and social-emotional domains in infant development. Even as very young infants, children are highly motivated to explore, gain information, attend, and engage their physical and social environments (Gibson 1987). As Gibson (1988, 5) explains: "We don't simply see, we look." Research by Berthier (1996, 811) indicates that "infant reaching is not simply a neural program that is triggered by the presence of a goal object, but that infants match the kinematics of their reaches to the task and their goals."

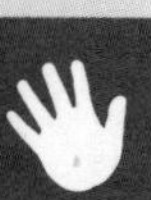

Perception and motor action play a key role in children's experiences and psychological processes (Thelen 1995). They also contribute to human psychological development in general, since ultimately "behavior is movement" (Adolph and Berger 2005, 223), and psychology can be defined as the study of human behavior. It has been proposed that infants' use of social information to guide their motor behavior in physically challenging or unfamiliar situations provides an excellent means to study infant social cognition (Tamis-LeMonda and Adolph 2005).

Perceptual Development

Infants' perceptual skills are at work during every waking moment. For example, those skills can be observed when an infant gazes into a caregiver's eyes or distinguishes between familiar and unfamiliar people. Infants use perception to distinguish features of the environment, such as height, depth, and color. "The human infant is recognized today as 'perceptually competent'; determining just how the senses function in infancy helps to specify the perceptual world of babies" (Bornstein 2005, 284). The ability to perceive commonalities and differences between objects is related to the cognitive domain foundation of classification. Infants explore objects differently depending upon object features such as weight, texture, sound, or rigidity (Palmer 1989). Parents and professionals may have observed young children exploring a slope, such as a slide, by touching it with their hands or feet before they decide whether to slide down it or not. Research by Adolph, Eppler, and Gibson (1993) suggests that learning plays a part in young children's decision making in physically risky situations, such as navigating slopes, and that exploratory behavior may be a means to this learning. Perception is also strongly related to the social-emotional domain, such as when young children perceive the differences between various facial expressions and come to understand what they may mean.

Gross Motor Development

Gross motor development includes the attainment of skills such as rolling over, sitting up, crawling, walking, and running. Gross motor behavior enables infants to move and thereby attain different and varied perspectives on the environment. Behaviors such as pulling to stand and climbing present children with new learning opportunities. When infants push a toy stroller or shopping cart, they are also engaging in processes related to cognitive development, such as imitation. The gross motor behaviors involved in active outdoor play with other children are related to children's development of social skills and an understanding of social rules.

Fine Motor Development

Through touching, grasping, and manual manipulation, infants experience a sense of agency and learn about the features of people, objects, and the environment. Fine motor development is related to the ability to draw, write, and participate in routines such as eating and dressing. Common early childhood learning materials, such as pegboards, stacking rings, stringing beads, and puzzles, offer opportunities for infants to practice their fine motor skills. Fine motor movements of the hands are coordinated with perceptual information provided through movements of the eyes, as when seven- to nine-month-old infants use visual information to orient their hands as they reach for an object (McCarty and others 2001).

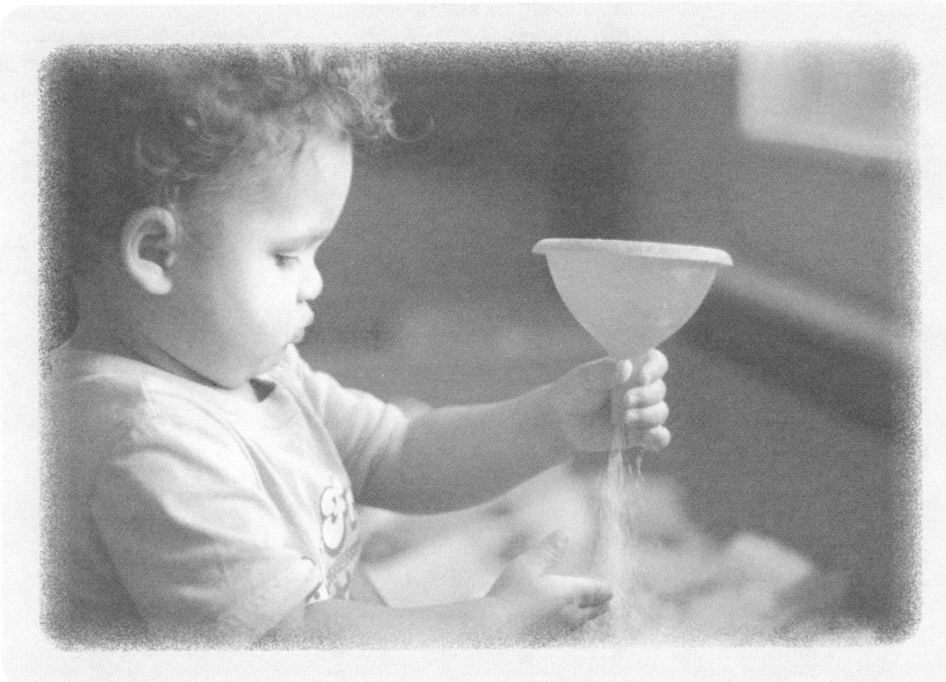

Foundation: Perceptual Development

The developing ability to become aware of the social and physical environment through the senses

8 months	*18 months*	*36 months*
At around eight months of age, children use the senses to explore objects and people in the environment. (6–9 mos.; Ruff and Kohler 1978)	At around 18 months of age, children use the information received from the senses to change the way they interact with the environment.	At around 36 months of age, children can quickly and easily combine the information received from the senses to inform the way they interact with the environment.
For example, the child may:	**For example, the child may:**	**For example, the child may:**
• Look at an object in her hand, mouth it, and then take it out to look at it again. (6–9 mos.; Ruff and Kohler 1978) • Hear the infant care teacher's footsteps in the darkened nap room and turn his head to try to look for her. (6–9 mos.; Ruff and Kohler 1978) • Show excitement upon recognizing the color of a favorite food that is offered on a spoon. (6–9 mos.; Reardon and Bushnell 1988)	• Adjust the way he is walking depending on the type of surface; for example, walking slowly on rocks and faster on pavement. (12–18 mos.; Fogel 2001, 333) • Choose to sit on her bottom and slide down a steep hill rather than walk down it. (12–18 mos.; Adolph, Eppler, and Gibson 1993) • Sway back and forth to the beat of a song while standing up. • Pull hands away from the sensory table, which is filled with an unfamiliar slimy substance. • Spend a lot of time in the sandbox, burying a hand underneath a pile of sand. • Stop pouring sand into a bucket that is already full.	• Identify a blanket or other familiar objects just by touching them. (30–36 mo.; Parks 2004) • Identify a truck when she feels it buried underneath the sand. (30–36 mos.; Parks 2004, 17) • Watch the lines that she makes with a marker on the paper. (Freeman 1980) • Climb more slowly as he reaches the top of the ladder. • Press harder on a clump of clay than on play dough. • Watch a family member draw a circle and then try to do it. (24–36 mos.; Stiles 1995) • Walk more slowly and carefully when carrying an open cup of milk than when carrying a cup with a lid.

Perceptual Development

Behaviors leading up to the foundation (4 to 7 months)	Behaviors leading up to the foundation (9 to 17 months)	Behaviors leading up to the foundation (19 to 35 months)
During this period, the child may: • Have a range of vision that is several feet. (By 4 mos.; American Academy of Pediatrics 2004, 207) • Experience the sensation of being touched, and then search for the object or person. (4–6 mos.; Parks 2004, 11) • Listen to the sounds that family members use while talking in the home language, and use these same sounds while babbling. (4–6 mos.; Parks 2004, 11) • Startle when hearing a loud noise. (By 4 mos.; American Academy of Pediatrics 2004, 209) • Kick feet while lying in the crib, feel the crib shake, and then kick feet again. (By 4 mos.; American Academy of Pediatrics 2004, 209) • Recognize an object as something she has seen before, even while looking at it from a different perspective. (By 4 mos.; Fogel 2001, 252) • Notice the difference between different songs that the infant care teacher sings. (By 6 mos.; Fogel 2001, 252) • Look confused upon hearing sounds that do not fit with the motions observed (for example, hearing a squeaking noise while seeing a rattle move). (By 6 mos.; Fogel 2001, 252) • Explore objects with the mouth. (By 7 mos.; American Academy of Pediatrics 2004, 208) • See different colors. (By 7 mos.; American Academy of Pediatrics 2004, 208) • See things from a distance. (By 7 mos.; American Academy of Pediatrics 2004, 208) • Track moving objects with both eyes together. (By 7 mos.; American Academy of Pediatrics 2004, 208)	During this period, the child may: • Nuzzle his face into a freshly washed blanket to smell it. (6–12 mos.; Parks 2004) • Show recognition of sounds, such as the mother's footsteps, water running in the bathtub, or the refrigerator door being opened. (18 mos.; Meisels and others 2003, 38) • Pat, push, mound, and squeeze play dough, experiencing all the ways it can be used. (18 mos.; Meisels and others 2003, 37) • Explore pegboard holes with a finger, then look around for something to fit in the holes. (18 mos.; Meisels and others 2003, 37) • Enjoy messy activities or show a dislike for messy activities. (12–18 mos.; Parks 2004, 14) • React to various sensations, such as extremes in temperature and taste. (12–18 mos.; Parks 2004, 14–15) • Crumple and tear paper. (7–9 mos.; Parks, 2004, 26) • Stop crawling when he reaches the edge of the couch. (By the time most infants are crawling; Walk and Gibson 1961) • Be able to remember where toys are stored in the classroom because she has crawled by them before. (By the time most infants are crawling; Bai and Bertenthal 1992; Campos and Bertenthal, 1989)	During this period, the child may: • Enjoy rough-and-tumble play. (18–24 mos.; Parks 2004, 16) • Handle fragile items carefully. (24–26 mos.; Parks 2004, 16) • Enjoy tactile books, such as books with faux fuzzy animal fur. (24–29 mos.; Parks 2004, 17) • Play with sand and water by filling up buckets, digging, and pouring water. (24–36 mos.; Parks 2004, 17)

Foundation: Gross Motor

The developing ability to move the large muscles

8 months	*18 months*	*36 months*
At around eight months of age, children demonstrate the ability to maintain their posture in a sitting position and to shift between sitting and other positions.	Around 18 months of age, children move from one place to another by walking and running with basic control and coordination.	At around 36 months of age, children move with ease, coordinating movements and performing a variety of movements.
For example, the child may:	**For example, the child may:**	**For example, the child may:**
• Sit on the floor, legs bent, with one leg closer to the body than the other. (8 mos.; Alexander, Boehme, and Cupps 1993, 134) • Use forearms to pull forward on the floor while on her tummy. (Scaled score of 9 for 7:16–8:15 mos.; Bayley 2006, 155) • Move from a sitting position onto hands and knees. (Scaled score of 10 for 7:16–8:15 mos.; Bayley 2006, 156)	• Stand on one foot, alone or with support. (Scaled score of 10 for 18:16–19:15 mos.; Bayley 2006, 163) • Walk sideways. (Scaled score of 10 for 18:16–19:15 mos.; Bayley 2006, 163) • Push a doll stroller or play shopping cart. (17–18.5 mos.; Parks 2004) • Climb onto an adult-sized couch. (By 18 mos.; Apfel and Provence 2001, 33) • Run. (Scaled score of 10 for 16:16–17:15 mos.; Bayley 2006, 162)	• Walk and run with skill, changing speed and direction. (36 mos.; Parks 2004; by 36 mos.; Davies 2004, 194). • Kick and throw a ball, but with little control of direction or speed. (36 mos.; Meisels and others 2003, 76) • Bend over to pick up a toy and stand up without trouble. (By 36 mos.; American Academy of Pediatrics 2004) • Pedal a tricycle. (32–36 mos.; Parks 2004; 36 mos.; Davies 2004, 194) • Climb up climbers and ladders. (34–36 mos.; Parks 2004) • Walk backward a few feet. (28–29.5 mos.; Parks 2004; scaled score of 10 for 34:16–35:15 mos.; Bayley 2006, #63, 167) • Jump up with both feet at the same time. (30–36 mos.; Parks 2004; by 30 mos.; Apfel and Provence 2001, 33) • Catch a medium-size ball. (35–36+ mos.; Parks 2004) • Walk up stairs, without holding on, placing one foot on each step. (30 mos.; Squires, Potter, and Bricker 1999; by end of 24–36 mos., 34–36+ mos.; Parks 2004, 304; scaled score of 10 for 35:16–36:15 mos.; Bayley 2006, 64)

Gross Motor

Behaviors leading up to the foundation (4 to 7 months)	Behaviors leading up to the foundation (9 to 17 months)	Behaviors leading up to the foundation (19 to 35 months)
During this period, the child may: • Hold onto a foot while lying on her back. (Scaled score of 10 for 5:16–6:15 mos.; Bayley 2006, 153) • Roll from back to stomach (4–6 mos.; Lerner and Ciervo 2003) • Roll from stomach to back. (4–6 mos.; Lerner and Ciervo 2003; Bayley 2006, 25; 5.38–7.5 mos.; Parks 2004) • Bring both hands to the mid-line while lying on his back. (16 weeks; Squires, Potter, and Bricker 1999) • Sit without support and turn to the left or right to reach an object. (Scaled score of 7 for 7:16–8:15 mos.; Bayley 2006, 154; 7 mos.; Mercer 1998, 243) • Balance on one side, bearing weight on the lower hip, arm, and leg, leaving the upper arm and leg free to move and to manipulate objects. (7 mos.; Alexander, Boehme, and Cupps 1993, 131–132). • Move from hands and knees into a sitting position. (7 mos.; Alexander, Boehme, and Cupps 1993, 135) • Rock on hands and knees, sometimes losing balance. (7 mos.; Alexander, Boehme, and Cupps 1993, 138)	During this period, the child may: • Creep on hands and knees or hands and feet. (By 9 mos.; Apfel and Provence 2001, 31) • Pull to a stand, using furniture for support. (Scaled score of 10 for 8:16–9:15 mos.; Bayley 2006, 157) • Cruise while holding onto furniture. (9.61–13 mos.; Parks 2004; scaled score of 10 for 9:16–10:15 mos.; Bayley 2006, 158) • Sit down from a standing position. (Scaled score of 9 for 10:16–11:15 mos.; Bayley 2006, 158) • Walk without support. (Scaled score of 9 for 12:16–13:15 mos.; Bayley 2006, 160; by 15 mos.; Apfel and Provence 2001, 33) • Throw a ball, underhand or overhand, to the infant care teacher. (Scaled score of 10 for 12:16–13:15 mos.; Bayley 2006, 160) • Squat to explore a toy on the ground and then stand up. (Scaled score of 10 for 13:16–14:15 mos.; Bayley 2006, 160) • Walk up or down stairs by stepping with both feet on each step while holding a parent's hand or the handrail. (Scaled score of 10 for up for 14:16–15:15 mos.; Bayley 2006, 161; for down for 15:16–16:15 mos.; Bayley 2006, 162) • Get into a standing position without support. (Around 11:15 mos.; Bayley 2006, 159) • Crawl or creep up or down a few steps.	During this period, the child may: • Jump off the bottom step. (24–26.5 mos.; Parks 2004; scaled score of 10 for 19:16–20:15 mos.; Bayley 2006, 164) • Kick a ball. (Scaled score of 10 for 20:16–21:15 mos.; Bayley 2006, 164; by 21 mos.; Apfel and Provence 2001, 33) • Ride a ride-on toy without pedals, pushing her feet on the ground to move. (18–24 mos.; Parks 2004) • Walk up or down stairs by stepping with both feet on each step, without holding on. (Scaled score of 10 for up for 24:16–25:15 mos.; Bayley 2006, 165) • Catch a big ball using two arms. (24–26+ mos.; Parks 2004) • Jump forward a few inches. (Scaled score of 10 for 27:16–28:15 mos.; Bayley 2006, 166) • Walk on tiptoes. (Scaled score of 10 for 32:16–33:15 mos.; Bayley 2006, 167; 36 mos.; Meisels and others 2003, 75)

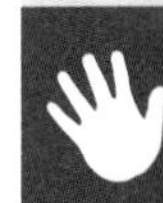

Foundation: Fine Motor

The developing ability to move the small muscles

8 months	*18 months*	*36 months*
At around eight months of age, children easily reach for and grasp things and use eyes and hands to explore objects actively. (6 mos.; Alexander, Boehme, and Cupps 1993, 112)	At around 18 months of age, children are able to hold small objects in one hand and sometimes use both hands together to manipulate objects. (18 mos.; Meisels and others 2003, 40)	At around 36 months of age, children coordinate the fine movements of the fingers, wrists, and hands to skillfully manipulate a wide range of objects and materials in intricate ways. Children often use one hand to stabilize an object while manipulating it.
For example, the child may:	**For example, the child may:**	**For example, the child may:**
• Reach for and grasp an object, using one hand. (5–8 mos.; *Introduction to Infant Development,* 2002, 62; by end of 7 mos.; American Academy of Pediatrics 2004, 205; 7–8 1/2 mos.; Parks 2004) • Use hand in a raking or sweeping motion to bring a toy closer. (7–8 mos.; Parks 2004; by end of 7 mos.; American Academy of Pediatrics 2004, 205; 7–8 mos.; Frankenburg and Dodds 1990) • Hold a small block using the thumb and fingertips. (item right before scaled score of 10 for 7:16–8:15 mos.; Bayley 2006, 127) • Hold a small block in each hand and bang the blocks together. (Scaled score of 10 7:16–8:15 mos.; Bayley 2006, 127)	• Hold a crayon between fingers and thumb. (13–18 mos.; Slater and Lewis 2002, 62; scaled score of 10 for 17:16–18:15 mos.; Bayley 2006, 131) • Scribble with big arm movements. (13–18 mos.; *Introduction to Infant Development,* 2002, 62) • Place pegs into a pegboard. (16–19 mos.; Parks 2004) • Hold a toy with one hand and use the fingers of the other hand to explore it. (By 18 mos.; Meisels and others 2003, 40) • Point to the pictures of a book. (By 18 mos.; Meisels and others 2003, 40) • Place a stacking ring on the post. (By 18 mos.; Meisels and others 2003, 40) • Use two hands to pick up a big truck, but only one hand to pick up a small one. (12–18 mos.; Parks 2004, 81) • Use the wrists to rotate objects in order to explore all sides. (18 mos.; Meisels and others 2003, 40) • Use one hand in opposition to the other. (18 mos.; Meisels and others 2003, 40)	• Use child-safe scissors in one hand to make snips in a piece of paper. (Scaled score of 10 for 34:16–35:15 mos.; Bayley 2006, 136; 28–35 mos.; Parks 2004) • String large wooden beads onto a shoelace. (33–36 mos.; Parks 2004) • Build a tall tower with six or more blocks. (28–31 mos.; Parks 2004; by the end of 24–36 mos.; American Academy of Pediatrics 2004, 305) • Turn the pages of a paper book, one at a time. (By end of 24–36 mos.; American Academy of Pediatrics 2004, 305) • Twist toy nuts and bolts on and off. (By end of 24–36 mos.; American Academy of Pediatrics 2004, 305) • Open a door by turning the round handle. (By end of 24–36 mos.; American Academy of Pediatrics 2004, 305) • Use one hand to hold and drink from a cup. (By 36 mos.; Meisels and others 2003, 77) • Place a wooden puzzle piece in the correct place in the puzzle. • Use thumb, index, and middle fingers to draw or write with a crayon, marker, or pencil. (Scaled score of 10 for 21:15–22:15 and 35:16–36:15 mos.; Bayley 2006, 136; by 36 mos.; Apfel and Provence 2001, 33)

Fine Motor

Behaviors leading up to the foundation (4 to 7 months)	Behaviors leading up to the foundation (9 to 17 months)	Behaviors leading up to the foundation (19 to 35 months)
During this period, the child may: • Transfer a cloth from one hand to another. (6 mos.; Alexander, Boehme, and Cupps 1993, 110; scaled score of 10 for 5:16–6:15 mos.; Bayley 2006) • Pull the spoon out of her mouth. (6 mos.; Alexander, Boehme, and Cupps 1993, 111) • Reach toward a toy and make grasping motions with the hand. (4–6 mos.; Lerner and Ciervo 2003) • Reach for a second toy when already holding one in the other hand. (5–6.5 mos.; Parks 2004, 49) • Hold one block in each hand, then drop one of them when the infant care teacher holds out a third block. (6.5–7.5 mos.; Parks 2004, 50) • Have the hands in an open position when relaxed. (4 mos.; Meisels and others 2003, 14)	During this period, the child may: • Hold on to two blocks while reaching for another block. (8–10 mos.; Parks 2004, 50) • Use thumb and index finger to pick up a piece of cereal. (Scaled score of 10 for 9:16–10:15 mos.; Bayley 2006, 128) • Drop a block into the wide opening of a large container. (9 mos.; Alexander, Boehme, and Cupps 1993, 157) • Turn the pages of a board book. (Scaled score of 10 for 9:16–10:15 mos.; Bayley 2006, 128) • Use hands to follow along with some motions of a song, chant, or finger play. (Scaled score of 10 for 9:16–10:15 mos.; Bayley 2006, 87) • Grasp onto and pull the string of a pull toy. (9–12 mos.; Parks 2004, 51) • Point with the index finger. (12 mos.; Coplan 1993, 3; scaled score of 10 for 11:16–12:15 mos.; Bayley 2006, 129) • Stack two to three small blocks into a tower. (Scaled score of 10 for 13:16–15:15 mos.; Bayley 2006, 130) • Unscrew the lid of a plastic jar. (Scaled score of 10 for 14:16–15:15 mos.; Bayley 2006, 62) • Put pieces of cereal inside a container with a small opening. (Scaled score of 10 for 16:16–17:15 mos.; Bayley 2006, 130)	During this period, the child may: • Fold a piece of paper. (21–24 mos.; Parks 2004) • Dump a container by turning it over. (By 24 mos.; American Academy of Pediatrics 2004) • Use a crayon to draw lines and circles on a piece of paper. (Scaled score of 10 for 27:16–28:15 mos.; Bayley 2006, 134; 30 mos.; Squires, Potter, and Bricker 1999; by 30 mos.; Apfel and Provence 2001, 33)

References

Adolph, K. E. 1997. "Learning in the Development of Infant Locomotion," *Monographs of the Society for Research in Child Development*, Vol. 62, No. 3, Serial No. 251.

Adolph, K. E. 2008. "Motor/Physical Development: Locomotion," in *Encyclopedia of Infant and Early Childhood Development*. Edited by M. M. Haith and J. B. Benson. San Diego, CA: Academic Press.

Adolph, K. E., and A. M. Avolio. 2000. "Walking Infants Adapt Locomotion to Changing Body Dimensions," *Journal of Experimental Psychology: Human Perception and Performance*, Vol. 26, No. 3, 1148–66.

Adolph, K. E., and S. E. Berger. 2005. "Physical and Motor Development," in *Developmental Science: An Advanced Textbook* (Fifth edition). Edited by M. H. Bornstein and M. E. Lamb. Hillsdale, NJ: Lawrence Erlbaum Associates.

Adolph, K. E., and S. E. Berger. 2006. "Motor Development," in *Handbook of Child Psychology: Volume 2: Cognition, Perception, and Language* (Sixth edition). Series Editors: W. Damon and R. Lerner. Volume Editors: D. Kuhn and others. New York: John Wiley and Sons.

Adolph, K. E.; M. A. Eppler; and E. J. Gibson. 1993. "Crawling Versus Walking Infants' Perception of Affordances for Locomotion over Sloping Surfaces," *Child Development*, Vol. 64, No. 4, 1158–74.

Adolph, K. E., and A. S. Joh. 2007. "Motor Development: How Infants Get Into the Act," in *Introduction to Infant Development* (Second edition). Edited by A. Slater and M. Lewis. New York: Oxford University Press.

Adolph, K. E.; B. Vereijken; and P. E. Shrout. 2003. "What Changes in Infant Walking and Why," *Child Development*, Vol. 74, No. 2, 475–97.

Adolph, K. E.; I. Weise; and L. Marin. 2003. "Motor Development," in *Encyclopedia of Cognitive Science*. London: Macmillan.

Alexander, R.; R. Boehme; and B. Cupps. 1993. *Normal Development of Functional Motor Skills*. San Antonio, TX: Therapy Skill Builders.

American Academy of Pediatrics. 2004. *Caring for Your Baby and Young Child: Birth to Age 5* (Fourth edition). Edited by S. P. Shelov and R. E. Hannemann. New York: Bantam Books.

Apfel, N. H., and S. Provence. 2001. *Manual for the Infant-Toddler and Family Instrument (ITFI)*. Baltimore: Brookes Publishing.

Bahrick, L. E.; R. Lickliter; and R. Flom. 2004. "Intersensory Redundancy Guides the Development of Selective Attention, Perception, and Cognition in Infancy," *Current Directions in Psychological Science*, Vol. 13, No. 3, 99–102.

Bai, D. L., and B. I. Bertenthal. 1992. "Locomotor Status and the Development of Spatial Search Skills," *Child Development*, Vol. 63, 215–26.

Bayley, N. 2006. *Bayley Scales of Infant and Toddler Development* (Third edition). San Antonio, TX: Harcourt Assessment.

Berthier, N. E. 1996. "Learning to Reach: A Mathematical Model," *Developmental Psychology*, Vol. 32, No. 5, 811–23.

Bertenthal, B. I. 1996. "Origins and Early Development of Perception, Action and Representation," *Annual Review of Psychology*, Vol. 47, 431–59.

Bertenthal, B. I., and S. M. Boker. 1997. "New Paradigms and New Issues: A Comment on Emerging Themes in the Study of Motor Development," *Monographs of the Society for Research in Child Development*, Vol. 62, No. 3, 141–51.

Bornstein, M. H. 2005. "Perceptual Development," in *Developmental Science: An Advanced Textbook* (Fifth edition). Edited by M. H. Bornstein and M. E. Lamb. Mahwah, NJ: Lawrence Erlbaum Associates.

Bushnell, E. W., and J. P. Boudreau. 1993. "Motor Development and the Mind: the Potential Role of Motor Abilities as a Determinant of Aspects of Perceptual Development," *Child Development,* Vol. 64, 1005–21.

Campos, J. J., and B. I. Bertenthal. 1989. "Locomotion and Psychological Development in Infancy" in *Applied Developmental Psychology.* Edited by F. Morrison, C. Lord, and D. Keating. New York: Academic Press.

Coplan, J. 1993. *Early Language Milestone Scale* (Second edition). Austin, TX: Pro-ed.

Davies, D. 2004. *Child Development: A Practitioner's Guide* (Second edition). New York: Guilford Press.

Diamond, A. 2007. "Interrelated and Interdependent," *Developmental Science,* Vol. 10, No. 1, 152–58.

Fogel, A. 2001. *Infancy: Infant, Family, and Society* (Fourth edition). Belmont, CA: Wadsworth/Thomson Learning.

Frankenburg, W. K., and others. 1990. *Denver II Screening Manual.* Denver, CO: Denver Developmental Materials.

Freeman, N. H. 1980. *Strategies of Representation in Young Children: Analysis of Spatial Skill and Drawing Processes.* London: Academic Press.

Gibson, E. J. 1987. "What Does Infant Perception Tell Us About Theories of Perception?" *Journal of Experimental Psychology: Human Perception and Performance,* Vol. 13, No. 4, 515–23.

Gibson, E. J. 1988. "Exploratory Behavior in the Development of Perceiving, Acting and the Acquiring of Knowledge," *Annual Review of Psychology,* Vol. 39, No. 1, 1–41.

Haith, M. M.; C. Hazen; and G. S. Goodman. 1988. "Expectation and Anticipation of Dynamic Visual Events by 3.5-Month-Old Babies," *Child Development,* Vol. 59, 467–79.

Introduction to Infant Development. 2002. Edited by A. Slater and M. Lewis. New York: Oxford University Press.

Lerner, C., and L. A. Ciervo. 2003. *Healthy Minds: Nurturing Children's Development from 0 to 36 Months.* Washington, DC: Zero to Three Press and American Academy of Pediatrics.

McCarty, M. E., and others. 2001. "How Infants Use Vision for Grasping Objects," *Child Development,* Vol. 72, No. 4, 973–87.

Meisels, S. J., and others. 2003. *The Ounce Scale: Standards for the Developmental Profiles* (Birth–42 Months). New York: Pearson Early Learning.

Mercer, J. 1998. *Infant Development: A Multidisciplinary Introduction.* Pacific Grove, CA: Brooks/Cole Publishing.

Palmer, C. F. 1989. "The Discriminating Nature of Infants' Exploratory Actions," *Developmental Psychology,* Vol. 25, No. 6, 885–93.

Parks, S. 2004. *Inside HELP: Hawaii Early Learning Profile: Administration and Reference Manual.* Palo Alto, CA: VORT Corporation.

Pick, H. L. 1989. "Motor Development: The Control of Action," *Developmental Psychology,* Vol. 25, No. 6, 867–70.

Reardon, P., and E. W. Bushnell. 1988. "Infants' Sensitivity to Arbitrary Pairings of Color and Taste," *Infant Behavior and Development,* Vol. 11, 245–50.

Ruff, H. A., and C. J. Kohler. 1978. "Tactual-Visual Transfer in Six-Month-Old Infants," *Infant Behavior and Development,* Vol. 1, 259–64.

Squires, J.; L. Potter; and D. Bricker. 1999. *The Ages and Stages Questionnaires User's Guide* (Second edition). Baltimore, MD: Paul H. Brookes Publishing.

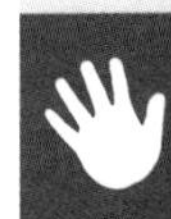

Stiles, J. 1995. "The Early Use and Development of Graphic Formulas: Two Case Study Reports of Graphic Formula Production by 2- to 3-Year Old Children," *International Journal of Behavioral Development,* Vol. 18, No. 1, 127–49.

Tamis-LeMonda, C. S., and K. E. Adolph. 2005. "Social Cognition in Infant Motor Action," in *The Development of Social Cognition and Communication.* Edited by B. Homer and C. S. Tamis-LeMonda. Mahwah, NJ: Lawrence Erlbaum Associates.

Thelen, E. 1994. "Three-Month-Old Infants Can Learn Task-Specific Patterns of Interlimb Coordination," *Psychological Science,* Vol. 5, No. 5, 280–85.

Thelen, E. 1995. "Motor Development: A New Synthesis," *American Psychologist,* Vol. 50, No. 2, 79–95.

Walk, R. D., and E. J. Gibson. 1961. "A Comparative and Analytic Study of Visual Depth Perception," *Psychological Monographs,* Vol. 75, No. 15.

von Hofsten, C. 2007. "Action in Development," *Developmental Science,* Vol. 10, No. 1, 54–60.

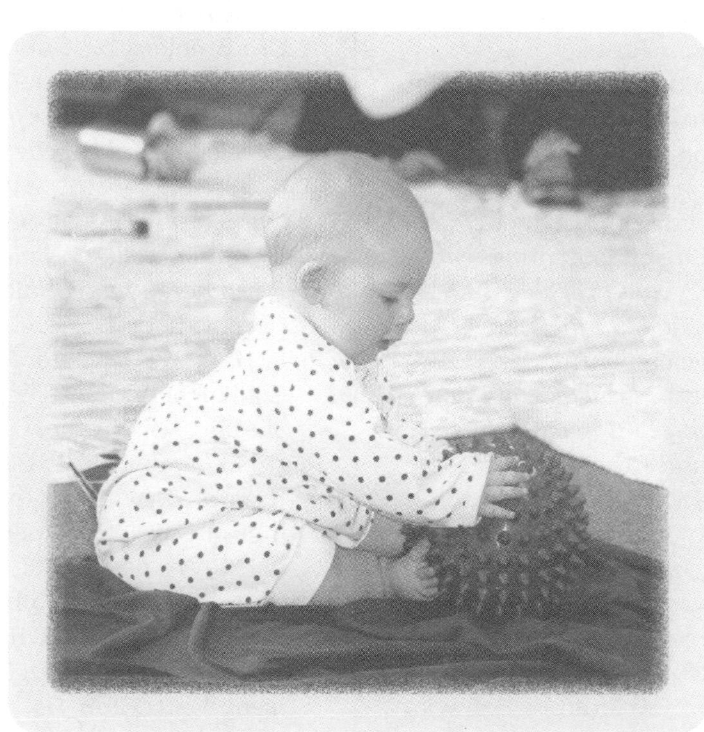

Appendix

Summary of Infant/Toddler Foundations

Social-Emotional Development

Interactions with Adults: The developing ability to respond to and engage with adults

Relationships with Adults: The development of close relationships with certain adults who provide consistent nurturance

Interactions with Peers: The developing ability to respond to and engage with other children

Relationships with Peers: The development of relationships with certain peers through interactions over time

Identity of Self in Relation to Others: The developing concept that the child is an individual operating within social relationships

Recognition of Ability: The developing understanding that the child can take action to influence the environment

Expression of Emotion: The developing ability to express a variety of feelings through facial expressions, movements, gestures, sounds, or words

Empathy: The developing ability to share in the emotional experiences of others

Emotion Regulation: The developing ability to manage emotional responses with assistance from others and independently

Impulse Control: The developing capacity to wait for needs to be met, to inhibit potentially hurtful behavior, and to act according to social expectations, including safety rules

Social Understanding: The developing understanding of the responses, communication, emotional expressions, and actions of other people

Language Development

Receptive Language: The developing ability to understand words and increasingly complex utterances

Expressive Language: The developing ability to produce the sounds of language and use vocabulary and increasingly complex utterances

Communication Skills and Knowledge: The developing ability to communicate nonverbally and verbally

Interest in Print: The developing interest in engaging with print in books and in the environment

Cognitive Development

Cause-and-Effect: The developing understanding that one event brings about another

Spatial Relationships: The developing understanding of how things move and fit in space

Problem Solving: The developing ability to engage in a purposeful effort to reach a goal or figure out how something works

Imitation: The developing ability to mirror, repeat, and practice the actions of others, either immediately or later

Memory: The developing ability to store and later retrieve information about past experiences

Number Sense: The developing understanding of number and quantity

Classification: The developing ability to group, sort, categorize, connect, and have expectations of objects and people according to their attributes

Symbolic Play: The developing ability to use actions, objects, or ideas to represent other actions, objects, or ideas

Attention Maintenance: The developing ability to attend to people and things while interacting with others and exploring the environment and play materials

Understanding of Personal Care Routines: The developing ability to understand and participate in personal care routines

Perceptual and Motor Development

Perceptual Development: The developing ability to become aware of the social and physical environment through the senses

Gross Motor: The developing ability to move the large muscles

Fine Motor: The developing ability to move the small muscles

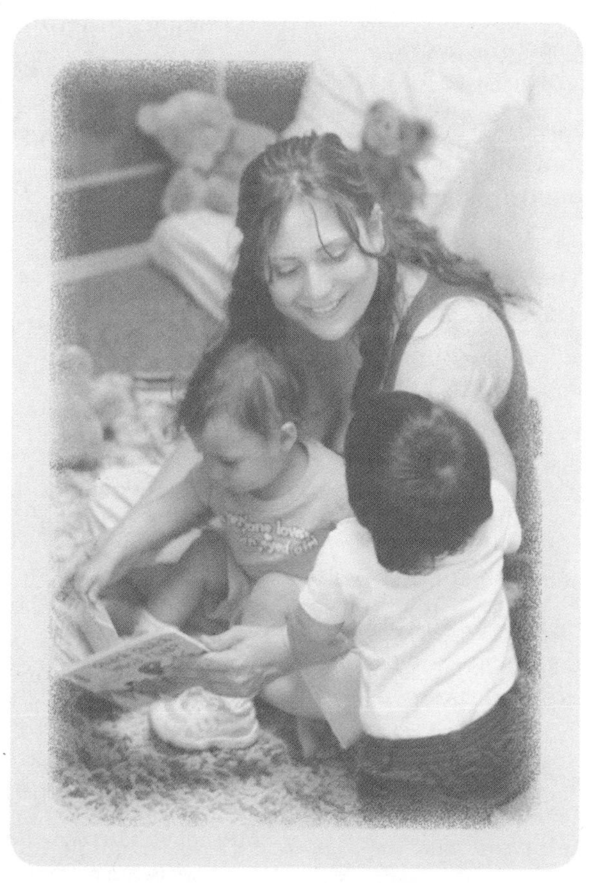

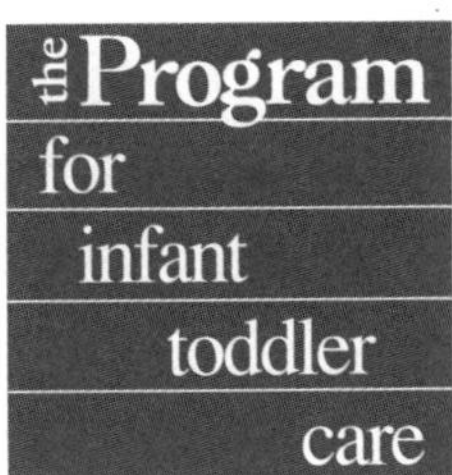

Price List and Order Form

MODULE I

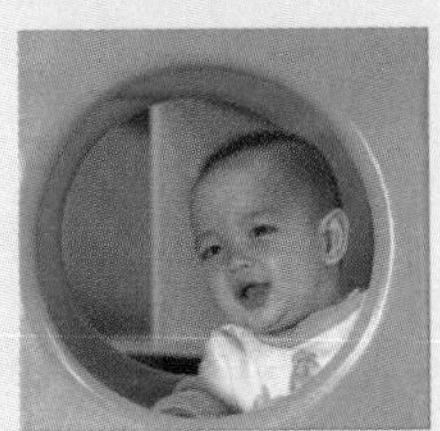

Social–Emotional Growth and Socialization

DVDs and Magazines

First Moves: Welcoming a Child to a New Caregiving Setting

Flexible, Fearful, or Feisty: The Different Temperaments of Infants and Toddlers

Getting in Tune: Creating Nurturing Relationships with Infants and Toddlers

Print Materials

Infant/Toddler Caregiving: A Guide to Social–Emotional Growth and Socialization

Module I Trainer's Manual

MODULE II

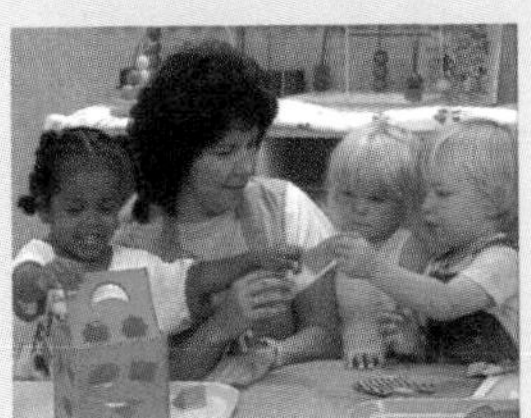

Group Care

DVDs and Magazines

It's Not Just Routine: Feeding, Diapering, and Napping Infants and Toddlers (Second edition)

Respectfully Yours: Magda Gerber's Approach to Professional Infant/ Toddler Care

Space to Grow: Creating a Child Care Environment for Infants and Toddlers (Second edition)

Together in Care: Meeting the Intimacy Needs of Infants and Toddlers in Groups

Print Materials

Infant/Toddler Caregiving: A Guide to Routines (Second edition)

Infant/Toddler Caregiving: A Guide to Setting Up Environments

Module II Trainer's Manual

MODULE III

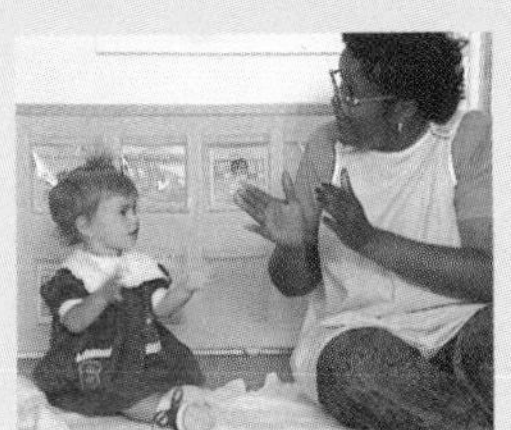

Learning and Development

DVDs and Magazines

The Ages of Infancy: Caring for Young, Mobile, and Older Infants

Discoveries of Infancy: Cognitive Development and Learning

Early Messages: Facilitating Language Development and Communication

The Next Step: Including the Infant in the Curriculum

Print Materials

Infant/Toddler Caregiving: A Guide to Cognitive Development and Learning

Infant/Toddler Caregiving: A Guide to Language Development and Communication

Module III Trainer's Manual

MODULE IV

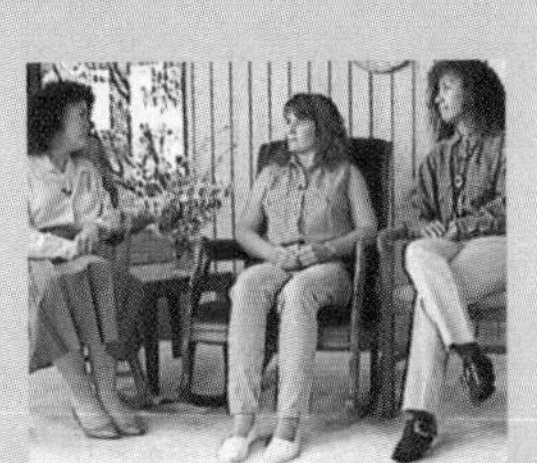

Culture, Family, and Providers

DVDs and Magazines

Essential Connections: Ten Keys to Culturally Sensitive Child Care

Protective Urges: Working with the Feelings of Parents and Caregivers

Print Materials

Infant/Toddler Caregiving: A Guide to Creating Partnerships with Families

Infant/Toddler Caregiving: A Guide to Culturally Sensitive Care

Module IV Trainer's Manual

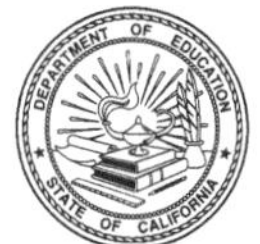

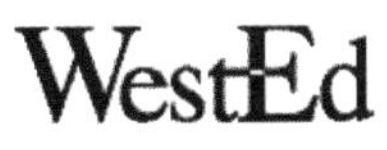

Each module includes DVDs, video magazines, curriculum guide(s), and a trainer's manual. All modules are available in English and Spanish. Additional PITC materials and new infant/ toddler items from the California Department of Education are listed on the last page of this order form.

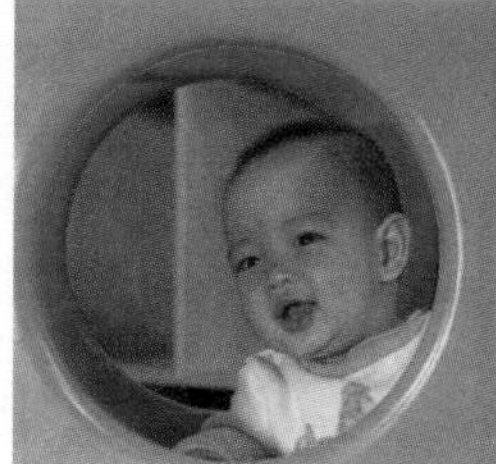

MODULE I
Social–Emotional Growth and Socialization

Title	Item no.	Quantity	Price	Total
Audiovisual Materials				
DVD (Each DVD includes a video magazine in the same language as the DVD.)				
First Moves (1988)	1636		$75.00	$
Los primeros pasos (1988)	1637		75.00	
Flexible, Fearful, or Feisty (1990)	1638		75.00	
Flexible, cauteloso, o inquieto (1990)	1639		75.00	
Getting in Tune (1990)	1644		75.00	
Llevar el compás (1990)	1645		75.00	
Print Materials				
Curriculum Guides				
A Guide to Social–Emotional Growth and Socialization (1990)	0876		$18.00	
Una guía para el crecimiento socioemocional y la socialización (2005)	1606		18.00	
Module I Trainer's Manual (1993)	1084		25.00	
Manual pedagógico, Módulo I: El crecimiento socioemocional y la socialización (2007)	1660		25.00	
Video Magazines (In packages of 50)				
First Moves - English	9960		$23.00	
First Moves - Spanish	9736		23.00	
Flexible, Fearful, or Feisty - English	9956		23.00	
Flexible, Fearful, or Feisty - Spanish	9737		23.00	
Getting in Tune - English	9957		23.00	
Getting in Tune - Spanish	9738		23.00	
MODULE I: SOCIAL–EMOTIONAL GROWTH AND SOCIALIZATION PACKAGE—$239				
Price includes 3 videos, 3 accompanying video magazines, 1 curriculum guide, and 1 trainer's manual.				
English DVDs/English guides/English manual	9696		**$239.00**	
Spanish DVDs/Spanish guides/Spanish manual	9695		**239.00**	
			SUBTOTAL	$

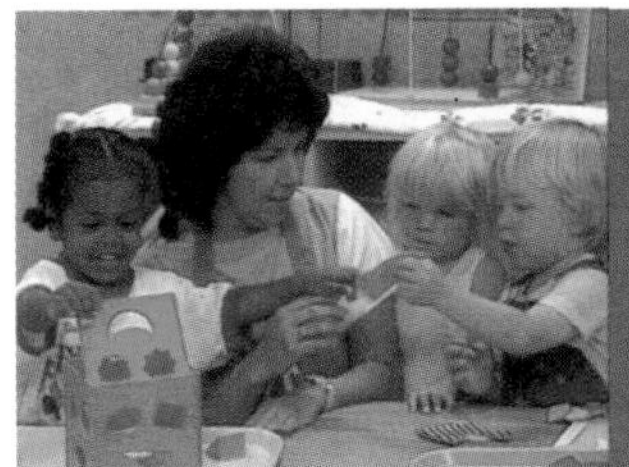

MODULE II
Group Care

Title	Item no.	Quantity	Price	Total
Audiovisual Materials				
DVD (Each DVD includes a video magazine in the same language as the DVD.)				
It's Not Just Routine (Second edition) (2000)	1648		$75.00	$
No es sólo una rutina (Segunda edición) (2000)	1649		75.00	
Respectfully Yours (1988)	1640		75.00	
Con respeto (1988)	1641		75.00	
Space to Grow (Second edition) (2004)	1646		75.00	
Un lugar para crecer (Segunda edición) (2004)	1647		75.00	
Together in Care (1992)	1632		75.00	
Unidos en el corazón (1992)	1633		75.00	
Print Materials				
Curriculum Guides				
A Guide to Routines (Second edition) (2000)	1510		$18.00	
Una guía para las rutinas cotidianas del cuidado infantil (Segunda edición) (2004)	1602		18.00	
A Guide to Setting Up Environments (1990)	0879		18.00	
Una guía para crear los ambientes del cuidado infantil (2006)	1614		18.00	
Module II Trainer's Manual (1993)	1076		25.00	
Manual pedagógico, Módulo II: El cuidado infantil en grupo (2007)	1661		25.00	
Video Magazines (In packages of 50)				
It's Not Just Routine (Second edition) - English	9724		$23.00	
It's Not Just Routine (Second edition) - Spanish	9723		23.00	
Respectfully Yours - English	9958		23.00	
Respectfully Yours - Spanish	9740		23.00	
Space to Grow (Second edition) - English	9709		23.00	
Space to Grow (Second edition) - Spanish	9710		23.00	
Together in Care - English	9873		23.00	
Together in Care - Spanish	9742		23.00	
MODULE II: GROUP CARE PACKAGE—$319				
Price includes 4 videos, 4 accompanying video magazines, 2 curriculum guides, and 1 trainer's manual.				
English DVDs/English guides/English manual	9694		**$319.00**	
Spanish DVDs/Spanish guides/Spanish manual	9693		**319.00**	
			SUBTOTAL	$

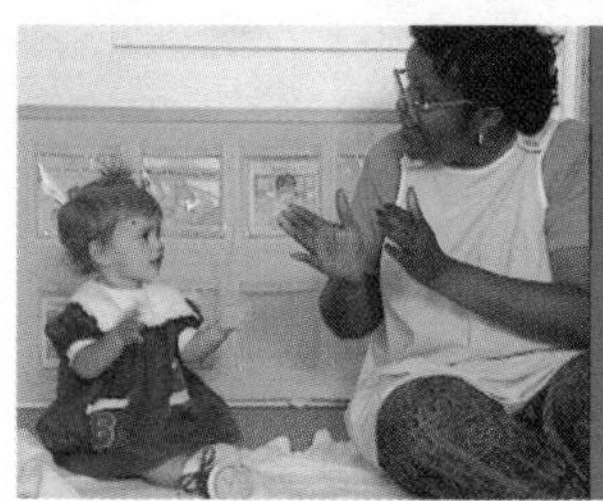

MODULE III
Learning and Development

Title	Item no.	Quantity	Price	Total
Audiovisual Materials				
DVD (Each DVD includes a video magazine in the same language as the DVD.)				
The Ages of Infancy (1990)	1634		$75.00	$
Las edades de la infancia (1990)	1635		75.00	
Discoveries of Infancy (1992)	1623		75.00	
Descubrimientos de la infancia (1992)	1624		75.00	
Early Messages (1998)	1625		75.00	
El comenzar de la comunicación (1998)	1626		75.00	
The Next Step (2004)	1621		75.00	
El siguiente paso (2004)	1622		75.00	
Print Materials				
Curriculum Guides				
A Guide to Cognitive Development and Learning (1995)	1055		$18.00	
Una guía para el desarrollo cognitivo y el aprendizaje (2006)	1616		18.00	
A Guide to Language Development and Communication (1990)	0880		18.00	
Una guía para el desarrollo del lenguaje y la comunicación (2006)	1608		18.00	
Module III Trainer's Manual (1993)	1108		25.00	
Manual pedagógico, Módulo III: Aprendizaje y desarrollo (2007)	1662		25.00	
Video Magazines (In packages of 50)				
The Ages of Infancy - English	9954		$23.00	
The Ages of Infancy - Spanish	9732		23.00	
Discoveries of Infancy - English	9874		23.00	
Discoveries of Infancy - Spanish	9733		23.00	
Early Messages - English	9747		23.00	
Early Messages - Spanish	9734		23.00	
The Next Step - English	9715		23.00	
The Next Step - Spanish	9697		23.00	
MODULE III: LEARNING AND DEVELOPMENT PACKAGE—$249				
Price includes 4 videos, 4 accompanying video magazines, 2 curriculum guides, and 1 trainer's manual.				
English DVDs/English guides/English manual	9692		**$249.00**	
Spanish DVDs/Spanish guides/English manual	9691		**249.00**	
			SUBTOTAL	$

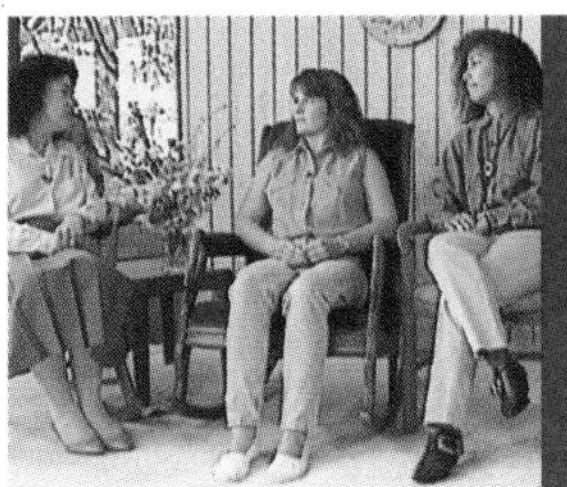

MODULE IV
Culture, Family, and Providers

Title	Item no.	Quantity	Price	Total
Audiovisual Materials				
DVD (Each DVD includes a video magazine in the same language as the DVD.)				
Essential Connections (1993)	1627		$75.00	$
Relaciones indispensables (1993)	1628		75.00	
Protective Urges (1996)	1630		75.00	
El instinto protector (1996)	1631		75.00	
Print Materials				
Curriculum Guides				
A Guide to Creating Partnerships with Families (1990)	0878		$18.00	
Una guía para establecer relaciones de colaboración con las familias (2006)	1615		18.00	
A Guide to Culturally Sensitive Care (1995)	1057		18.00	
Una guía para el cuidado infantil culturalmente sensible (2006)	1617		18.00	
Module IV Trainer's Manual (1995)	1109		25.00	
Manual pedagógico, Módulo IV: La cultura, la familia y los proveedores (2007)	1663		25.00	
Video Magazines (In packages of 50)				
Essential Connections - English	9869		$23.00	
Essential Connections - Spanish	9735		23.00	
Protective Urges - English	9778		23.00	
Protective Urges - Spanish	9739		23.00	
MODULE IV: CULTURE, FAMILY, AND PROVIDERS PACKAGE—$189				
Price includes 2 videos, 2 accompanying video magazines, 2 curriculum guides, and 1 trainer's manual.				
English DVDs/English guides/English manual	9690		**$189.00**	
Spanish DVDs/Spanish guides/Spanish manual	9689		**189.00**	
Supplemental Materials to Module IV				
DVD (Each DVD includes a video magazine.)				
Talking Points for Essential Connections - English (1998)	1643		$35.00	
Talking Points for Protective Urges - English (1998)	1642		25.00	
Video Magazines (In packages of 50)				
Talking Points for Essential Connections - English	9744		$23.00	
Talking Points for Protective Urges - English	9743		23.00	
			SUBTOTAL	$

Additional Materials

Title	Item no.	Quantity	Price	Total
Audiovisual Materials				
DVD (includes a video magazine) In Our Hands - English (1997)	1629		$25.00	$
Print Materials				
Addendum to Trainer's Manuals I, II, III, IV: Spanish Handouts/Transparencies (Second edition)	1679		$25.00	
The Family Child Care Supplement to Trainer's Manuals	7096		25.00	
Video Magazine (In packages of 50) In Our Hands - English (1997)	9749		23.00	
Materials from the California Department of Education				
Infant/Toddler Learning and Development: Program Guidelines (2006)	1619		$19.95	
New Perspectives (DVD) (2007)	1665		29.00	
			SUBTOTAL	$
			California residents add sales tax.	
			Shipping and handling charges (See chart.)	
			TOTAL	$

To order call: 1-800-995-4099

BUSINESS HOURS: 8:00 A.M.–4:30 P.M., PST, MONDAY THROUGH FRIDAY

NAME/ATTENTION

ADDRESS

CITY STATE ZIP CODE

COUNTY ( ) DAYTIME TELEPHONE

PAYMENT METHOD:

☐ CHECK (Payable to California Department of Education)

☐ VISA

☐ MASTERCARD

☐ PURCHASE ORDER

CREDIT CARD NUMBER

EXPIRATION DATE

AUTHORIZED SIGNATURE

SHIPPING CHARGES

Number of Items	
1–50	$4.95 per order plus $1.00 per item
51+	Call 1-800-995-4099 for discounted rate

All orders to be delivered within the continental United States are shipped via ground service unless expedited shipping is requested.

Additional charges apply on shipments to Alaska and Hawaii.

Note: Shipping and handling charges for modules are $5.95 for each module.

Visit our Web site: **http://www.cde.ca.gov/re/pn**

☐ **Please send me a free copy of the current Educational Resources Catalog.**

Mail completed order form to:

California Department of Education
CDE Press Sales Office
1430 N Street, Suite 3207
Sacramento, CA 95814-5901

Note: Mail orders must be accompanied by a check, a purchase order, or a VISAor MasterCard credit card number, including expiration date and your signature. Purchase orders without checks are accepted from educational institutions, businesses, and governmental agencies. Purchase orders may be placed by faxing to (916) 323-0823. Telephone orders will be accepted toll-free (1-800-995-4099) for credit card purchases. Please do not send cash. Stated prices are subject to change. Please order carefully; include correct item number and quantity for each publication ordered. **All sales are final.**

OSP 09 112060 08-002 PR070082-00 1-09 77M